# Radiology

*Guest Editor*

KATHLEEN A. GROSS, MSN, RN-BC, CRN

# PERIOPERATIVE NURSING CLINICS

www.periopnursing.theclinics.com

*Consulting Editor*
NANCY GIRARD, PhD, RN, FAAN

June 2010 • Volume 5 • Number 2

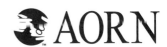

SAUNDERS an imprint of ELSEVIER, Inc.

## W.B. SAUNDERS COMPANY

*A Division of Elsevier Inc.*

1600 John F. Kennedy Boulevard • Suite 1800 • Philadelphia, Pennsylvania 19103-2899

http://www.periopnursing.theclinics.com

**PERIOPERATIVE NURSING CLINICS Volume 5, Number 2**
**June 2010 ISSN 1556-7931, ISBN-13: 978-1-4377-1858-4**

Editor: Katie Hartner
Developmental Editor: Donald Mumford

*Perioperative Nursing Clinics* (ISSN 1556-7931) is published quarterly by Elsevier, 360 Park Avenue South, New York, NY 10010. Months of issue are March, June, September and December. Business and Editorial Offices: 1600 John F. Kennedy Blvd., Suite 1800, Philadelphia, PA 19103-2899. Customer Service Office: 11830 Westline Industrial Drive, St. Louis, MO 63146. Periodicals postage paid at New York, NY and at additional mailing offices. Subscription prices are $116.00 per year (domestic individuals), $213.00 per year (domestic institutions), $58.00 per year (domestic students/residents), $150 per year (international individuals), $245 per year (international institutions), and $62.00 per year (International students/residents). Foreign air speed delivery is included in all *Clinics* subscription prices. All prices are subject to change without notice. **POSTMASTER:** Send change of address to *Perioperative Nursing Clinics*, Customer Service (orders, claims, online, change of address): Elsevier Periodicals Customer Service, 11830 Westline Industrial Drive, St. Louis, MO 63146. Tel: 1-800-654-2452 (U.S. and Canada). Fax: 314-523-5170. E-mail: journalscustomerservice-usa@elsevier.com (for print support); journalsonlinesupport-usa@elsevier.com (for online support).

*Reprints.* For copies of 100 or more, of articles in this publication, please contact the Commercial Rights Department, Elsevier Inc., 360 Park Avenue South, New York, NY 10010-1710; phone: (+1) 212-633-3813; fax: (+1) 212-462-1935; e-mail: reprints@elsevier.com.

Printed in the United States of America.

# Contributors

## CONSULTING EDITOR

**NANCY GIRARD, PhD, RN, FAAN**
Consultant, Boerne; Clinical Associate Professor, Acute Nursing Care Department, University of Texas Health Science Center, San Antonio, Texas

## GUEST EDITOR

**KATHLEEN A. GROSS, MSN, RN-BC, CRN**
Owings Mills, Maryland

## AUTHORS

**JAMES G. CARIDI, MD, FSIR**
Associate Professor of Radiology and Pediatrics, Chief of Vascular and Interventional Radiology, Shands Hospital, University of Florida College of Medicine, Gainesville, Florida

**DEBRA DENNY, RN, MHA**
Manager of Quality and Compliance, Baptist Cardiac and Vascular Institute, Baptist Hospital of Miami, Miami, Florida

**CAROL ELIADI, APRN, EdD, JD**
Associate Professor and Chief Nursing Officer, Department of Nursing, School of Nursing, Massachusetts College of Pharmacy and Health Sciences-Worcester, Worcester, Massachusetts

**CAROLYN J. FRIEL, RPh, PhD**
Associate Professor of Medicinal Chemistry, Department of Pharmaceutical Sciences, School of Pharmacy, Massachusetts College of Pharmacy and Health Sciences-Worcester, Worcester, Massachusetts

**JEFFREY P. GONZALES, PharmD, BCPS**
Assistant Professor, Critical Care, Department of Pharmacy Practice and Science, University of Maryland School of Pharmacy, Baltimore, Maryland

**CINDY GRINES, MD, FACC, FSCAI**
Department of Cardiovascular Medicine, William Beaumont Hospital, Royal Oak, Michigan

**MARION L. GROWNEY, MSN, ACNP**
Acute Care Nurse Practitioner, NeuroInterventional Radiology, Massachusetts General Hospital, Massachusetts

**STEPHEN B. HAUG, RTR, CV**
Program Director, Tegtmeyer School of Angio/Interventional Radiology, Division of Radiology, University of Virginia Health System, Charlottesville, Virginia

**IRVIN F. HAWKINS, MD, FSIR**
Professor of Radiology and Surgery, University of Florida College of Medicine, Shands Hospital, Gainesville, Florida

**JOSHUA A. HIRSCH, MD**
Vice Chief, Interventional Radiology; Director, NeuroInterventional Radiology/Endovascular Neurosurgery; Chief, Minimally Invasive Spine Surgery, Massachusetts General Hospital; Associate Professor, Harvard Medical School, Boston, Massachusetts

**BARRY T. KATZEN, MD**
Medical Director and Founder, Baptist Cardiac and Vascular Institute, Baptist Hospital of Miami, Miami, Florida

**JANE KIAH, RN, MS**
Director of Cardiac and Vascular Services, Baptist Cardiac and Vascular Institute, Baptist Hospital of Miami, Miami, Florida

**LOU-ELLEN LALLIER, MS, CRNP**
Acute Care Nurse Practitioner, Medical Intensive Care Unit, University of Maryland Medical Center, Baltimore, Maryland

**JAIME LEE, BSN, MSN, ARNP**
Nurse Practitioner, Interventional Radiology Department, Georgetown University Hospital, Washington, DC

**ALAN H. MATSUMOTO, MD, FSIR, FACR**
Professor of Angiography, Interventional Radiology and Special Procedures, Chair, Division of Radiology, Director, University of Virginia Core Lab and Clinical Over Road Service, University of Virginia Health System, Charlottesville, Virginia

**SANDRA OLIVER-MCNEIL, RN, MSN, ACNP-BC**
Department of Cardiovascular Medicine, William Beaumont Hospital, Royal Oak, Michigan

**KIMBERLY A. PESATURO, PharmD, BCPS**
Assistant Professor of Pharmacy Practice, Department of Pharmacy Practice, School of Pharmacy, Massachusetts College of Pharmacy and Health Sciences-Worcester, Worcester, Massachusetts

**GAIL EGAN SANSIVERO, MS, ANP**
Nurse Practitioner, Interventional Radiology, Community Care Physicians, PC, Latham; Instructor, Department of Radiology, Albany Medical College, Albany, New York

**SANDRA L. SCHWANER, MSN, ACNP-BC**
Acute Care Nurse Practitioner, APN1 Department of Interventional Radiology, Division of Radiology, University of Virginia Health System; Department of Radiology, Division of Interventional Radiology, Charlottesville, Virginia

**DEBBIE SMITH, RN, BSN, CNOR**
Perioperative Clinical Nurse Specialist, Clinical Learning, Baptist Health South Florida, Miami, Florida

**MELANIE STOIA, RN, BSN**
Chair, Shared Governance Committee, Interventional Services, Baptist Cardiac and Vascular Institute, Baptist Hospital of Miami, Miami, Florida

**RICHARD J. VETTER, PhD**
Professor of Biophysics, Division of Preventive, Occupational and Aerospace Medicine; Director of Occupational Safety, Radiation Safety Office, Mayo Clinic, Rochester, Minnesota

# Contents

in technology have led to particles and coils that can compress to travel through microcatheters and then expand to occlude the lumen of the vessel once released. Greater control of coils and particles also reduces the side effects of nontarget embolization and tissue necrosis. Advances in glue and in the use of temporary agents such as Gelfoam have also increased the number of applications available. Procedures can be performed in a planned, controlled environment, in conjunction with surgery, or emergently. Side effects include postembolization syndrome, infection, bleeding and/or hematoma, and abscess or necrosis of organ or tissue. Nursing management in the periprocedural period is essential. The nurse has an important role in evaluation of laboratory values and overall patient condition before, during, and after the procedure as well as patient education regarding what to expect.

$CO_2$ digital subtraction angiography can be used as an alternative or adjunct to iodinated contrast in vascular imaging and interventional procedures. Its unique qualities make it useful in diagnostic as well as therapeutic procedures in arteries and veins. Because of its endogenous gaseous attributes, it is nonallergic, does not affect the kidneys, and can be used in unlimited quantities. Compared with iodinated contrast, the low viscosity of $CO_2$ permits greater sensitivity for arterial hemorrhage and arteriovenous fistulas as well as the more facile use in microcatheters. Certain simple principles must be used with $CO_2$ as an imaging agent. When used appropriately, $CO_2$ is safe and can be useful when iodinated contrast is either not sufficient or is contraindicated.

The postoperative or bedside nurse is usually the first health care member to observe the subtle initial changes that a patient exhibits in early sepsis. This review provides an evidence-based approach for the acute management of sepsis and severe sepsis, focusing primarily on the initial critical hours. Topics reviewed include evaluation and diagnosis of sepsis, fluid resuscitation, antibiotic therapy, source control, and vasopressors/inotropic agents.

Local anesthesia is a pharmacologic technique used to render a small part of the body insensitive to pain. It allows the patient to safely undergo select medical or surgical procedures with reduced pain without altering their level of consciousness. Local anesthesia may also be used before venous cannulation, lumbar puncture, skin suturing, or to prevent pain caused by bone and/or muscle manipulations. This article reviews the physiology of pain, the mechanism of action and chemistry of the local anesthetics, adverse reactions, common dosages, and special considerations for the perioperative nurse managing patients receiving local anesthetics. This article also supplements the published AORN recommended practices for managing the patient receiving local anesthesia.

The benefits of hybrid operating suites are well documented. At Baptist Cardiac and Vascular Institute, the utility, safety and effectiveness of a hybrid interventional radiology suite continues to be demonstrated with optimal patient outcomes for endovascular aneurysm repair procedures. This article describes the redesign and upgrades to the suite, operational and cost efficiency measures implemented, and the creation of a team of highly competent hybrid staff.

Uterine fibroids are benign tumors of the myometrium that are found in 70% to 80% of all women of reproductive age, most of whom remain asymptomatic. Although they are benign, uterine fibroids are often the cause of severe symptoms including menorrhagia (heavy menstrual bleeding) and anemia, as well as bulk-related symptoms such as pain (pelvic, low back, flank, legs), pelvic pressure, abdominal bloating and increased girth, urinary symptoms (frequency, urgency, nocturia, incontinence, ureteral compression leading to hydronephrosis), and constipation. For the 20% to 30% of women who do present with any of these symptoms, it is imperative that a comprehensive work up be done, as many symptoms can also have other medical diagnoses. If uterine fibroids are diagnosed, all appropriate therapeutic options including medical therapies, surgical therapies (myomectomy, hysterectomy, and uterine fibroid embolization), and watchful waiting should be presented, and discussed, with the patient.

Vertebral compression fractures cause a substantial amount of morbidity and mortality. Fractures may be related to osteoporosis or a malignancy. Medical management in the forms of bedrest, bracing, and narcotic pain management is not a risk-free option. Vertebral augmentation, including vertebroplasty and kyphoplasty, is a minimally invasive option during which cement is placed into the fractured vertebra resulting in marked pain improvement. In the elderly population and among oncology patients, quality of life is of paramount importance. Vertebral augmentation offers a method of reducing pain and restoring independence for our most vulnerable patients.

**THE CLINICS ARE NOW AVAILABLE ONLINE!**
Access your subscription at:
**www.theclinics.com**

# Preface

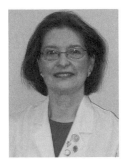

Kathleen A. Gross, MSN, RN-BC, CRN
*Guest Editor*

It has been my goal as Guest Editor to present a variety of subjects in the area of interventional radiology that would not only be of interest but valuable, practically, to perioperative nurses. Only you, the reader, can judge whether I have achieved that goal. I hope this issue exceeds your expectations. This issue of *Perioperative Nursing Clinics* would not have been possible without the hard work of all the authors. To each and every one, I truly owe a debt of thanks for their willingness to take on the task of preparing a timely manuscript and time away from their personal lives. They are all dedicated professionals who have helped share my vision for this issue.

Interventional radiology (IR) is a relatively new specialty in the spectrum of medicine and surgery. Historically, much of the work of IR involved diagnostic vascular procedures. Today IR is not only involved in the diagnosis but also the treatment of vascular and nonvascular diseases. In my career as an interventional radiology nurse, I have seen some procedures decline in use in favor of newer technologies, (eg, routine diagnostic cerebral angiography for carotid disease being replaced by CT or MRI imaging) and other procedures emerge as important advances in the field (eg, uterine artery embolization as an important alternative for some women with uterine fibroids). This dynamic aspect makes interventional radiology a unique area. Interventional radiology takes pride in offering minimally invasive options for a variety of medical problems. Today some interventional procedures incorporate the use of more than one imaging modality for a procedure.

Technological advances, more complex procedures, and patient acuity have impacted the nursing needs of the patient. Nurses are indispensible given the interventional radiology patients' needs. There are so many opportunities for nurses to pioneer nursing care for new procedures, to create new policies, and to set new standards in interventional radiology. Learning takes place everyday. It is an exciting area in which to work. Working in interventional radiology means that the registered nurse is part of a team including radiologists, technologists, anesthesia providers, physicists, pharmacists, administrative staff, and other personnel. This aspect of interventional radiology is reflected in the diversity of the authors who contributed to this issue.

Perioperative Nursing Clinics 5 (2010) xi–xii
doi:10.1016/j.cpen.2010.04.001
1556-7931/10/$ – see front matter © 2010 Elsevier Inc. All rights reserved.

**periopnursing.theclinics.com**

Interventional radiology procedures are not only taking place in interventional radiology suites. They also take place within the operating room or a free standing imaging facility. For this reason it is imperative that knowledge of interventional radiology nursing be shared with nursing colleagues from other specialities. Peri-anesthesia care nurses may be involved in patient preparation and recovery of the patient following an interventional procedure. The nurse is the healthcare provider who is most accessible to the patient during the continuum of care, as an outpatient or inpatient. The nurse is there to assess, evaluate, communicate, provide care, and teach patients and their significant other.

It has been my pleasure to work on this issue of *Perioperative Nursing Clinics.* Accepting new challenges has always been something I like to do. I have learned so much in the process and met so many wonderful people. I wish to thank Nancy Girard, PhD, RN, FAAN, Consulting Editor, for her guidance and support throughout the past months. Again, my sincerest thanks to all the contributing authors. To all the readers, please enjoy and learn from this issue.

Kathleen A. Gross, MSN, RN-BC, CRN
Owings Mills, MD, USA

E-mail address:
rgross@comcast.net

# Contrast-induced Nephropathy: Acute Kidney Injury

Sandra Oliver-McNeil, RN, MSN, ACNP-BC*,
Cindy Grines, MD, FSCAI

KEYWORDS

• Contrast • Osmolarity • Meta-analysis • Mortality

Contrast agents are indicated in cardiac catheterization laboratories without risk of causing acute kidney injury (AKI) in most patients. However, patients who develop contrast-induced AKI (CI-AKI) have an increased risk of long-term morbidity and mortality. Research to prevent AKI has been conducted to identify patients at increased risk and strategies to limit the injury. Strategies to minimize acute renal injury have been identified, including the administration of 0.9 normal saline (NS) and N-acetylcysteine, limiting the amount of contrast for procedures, and avoiding multiple exposures to contrast. The purpose of this article is to identify patients at risk and review strategies that can be used to prevent AKI.

## CONTRAST AGENTS

Contrast agents are classified into high-osmolar contrast media (HOCM) and low-osmolar contrast media (LOCM). Osmolarity of contrast is determined by the chemical structure of the agent. LOCM is divided into high-viscosity contrast medium and low-viscosity contrast medium. The higher the osmolarity, the longer the agent takes to clear the kidneys, thus increasing the risk of AKI.[1] The lower osmolarity of the nonionic agents may have an increased incidence of catheter thrombosis.

The HOCM include diatrizoate and iothalamate. The osmolality of the agents ranges from 2016 to 1400 mOsm/kg $H_2O$ compared with normal serum osmolality of 280 to 300 mOsm/kg $H_2O$. The LOCM with high viscosity are nonionic dimer such as iodixanol and nonionic monomers such as iopromide, iopamidol, iohexol, ioversol, and ioxilan. The osmolality of these agents are significantly less than HOCM, ranging from 844 to 290 mOsm/kg $H_2O$ (**Table 1**).[1] The risk of total adverse reactions for HOCM is 12.66% versus 3.13% for LOCM, with a P value of less than 0.01 (**Table 2**). Most adverse events for HOCM are short lived and benign (electrocardiographic changes,

Department of Cardiovascular Medicine, William Beaumont Hospital, 3601 West 13 Mile Road, Royal Oak, MI 48073, USA
* Corresponding author.
E-mail address: Sandra.Olivermcneil@beaumonthospitals.com

Perioperative Nursing Clinics 5 (2010) 101–110
doi:10.1016/j.cpen.2010.02.010
1556-7931/10/$ – see front matter © 2010 Elsevier Inc. All rights reserved.
periopnursing.theclinics.com

**Table 1**
**Classification of select contrast media used for cardiac procedures**

|  | Class | Chemical Name | Trade Name | Osmolality (mOsm/kg H$_2$O) | Viscosity (mPas at 20°C) |
|---|---|---|---|---|---|
| HOCM | Ionic monomers | Diatrizoate | Hypaque | 2016 | n/a |
|  |  |  | RenoCal-76 | 1870 | n/a |
|  |  |  | MD-76R | 1551 | n/a |
|  |  | Iothalamate | Conray | 1400 | n/a |
| (LOCM) High-viscosity contrast medium (HVCM) | Nonionic dimer | Iodixanol | Visipaque 320 | 290 | 26.6 |
|  | Nonionic monomers | Iopromide | Utravist 370 | 774 | 22.0 |
|  |  | Iopamidol | Isovue 370 | 796 | 20.9 |
|  |  | Iohexol | Omnipaque 350 | 844 | 20.4 |
|  |  | Ioversol | Optiray 350 | 792 | 18.0 |
|  |  | Ioxilan | Oxilan 350 | 695 | 16.3 |
| Low-viscosity contrast medium (LVCM) | Ionic dimer | Ioxaglate | Hexabrix 320 | 600 | 13.7 |

bradycardia, nausea, and hives) but may also include AKI with 20% increase in creatinine level, with anaphylaxis and very severe adverse reactions occurring in less than 1% of HOCM (see **Table 2**).

## RISK OF CLOTTING

The concerns with the use of contrast material include the risk of clotting during the procedure. In vitro clots form in static blood mixed with contrast. Nonionic agents have less anticoagulant properties and less antiplatelet effects compared with ionic contrast. The viscosity of contrast may alter flow patterns and shear forces. Two randomized trials in the 1990s compared low osmolar ionic contrast with nonionic contrast in acute myocardial infarction or unstable angina. The first study from William Beaumont Hospital, Royal Oak showed that the use of ionic LOCM reduced the risk of ischemic complications acutely and at 1 month after procedures.[2] This reduced risk supported the use of LOCM in the highest-risk group for thrombosis.

After 1999, there was increased use of potent antithrombin and antiplatelet agents during coronary interventions; thus, later studies showed no difference in thrombotic events between ionic and nonionic agents. This was likely due to maintaining therapeutic activated clotting time during the procedure, routine use of clopidogrel before the

**Table 2**
**Adverse reactions to contrast media**

|  | HOCM | LOCM | P Value |
|---|---|---|---|
| Total adverse reactions | 12.66% | 3.13% | <0.01 |
| Severe adverse reactions | 0.22% | 0.04% | <0.01 |
| Very severe adverse reactions[a] | 0.04% | 0.004% | <0.01 |

[a] Requiring anesthesia or hospitalization.

procedure, and the use of glycoprotein IIb/IIIa agents. The risk of increasing thrombosis with nonionic LOCM is probably neutralized with the use of other antithrobotic therapies. Future challenges will be to balance the risk of bleeding versus the risk of clotting.

## RISK FACTORS FOR DEVELOPING CI-AKI

Several risks have been identified that increase the risk for CI-AKI (**Box 1**).[3] Preexisting risks include underlying chronic renal disease and diabetes mellitus (DM). Decrease in estimated glomerular filtration rate (eGFR) increases the risk of CI-AKI. As the eGFR becomes less than 60mL/min, the risk of CI-AKI significantly increases.[4] The risk of CI-AKI increases from less than 10% with an eGFR of 60mL/min to 30% with an eGFR of less than 40 mL/min. DM without renal disease increases the risk by 4 fold with the administration of contrast material. If a patient has DM and renal disease, the risk of 1-year mortality increases to 25.9%.[5]

As the amount of contrast volume increases, so does the risk of contrast-induced nephropathy (CIN).[6] Moreover, arterial route of administration has a 50% increase in risk of CI-AKI compared with intravenous contrast.[7]

Lower hematocrit levels increase at baseline the risk of CI-AKI. Hematocrit levels of less than 36.7% have a 23.3% increased risk of developing CI-AKI.[8] The cause is unknown, but the possibility that the patient has underlying renal disease or dehydration as a result of blood loss may be the cause.

Other risk factors include underlying renal insufficiency; DM; age; volume depletion; hypotension; low cardiac output; congestive heart failure (CHF); hypoalbuminemia;

---

**Box 1**
**Risk factors for CIN**

*Patient-related risk factors*

- Renal insufficiency
- DM
- Age
- Volume depletion
- Hypotension
- Low cardiac output, CHF
- Hypoalbuminemia (<35 g/L)
- Anemia
- Renal transplant
- Other nephrotoxins (NSAIDs, cyclosporine, aminoglycosides, furosemide)

*Procedure-related risk factors*

- Multiple contrast media injection within 72 hours
- Intra-arterial injection site
- High volume of contrast media
- High osmolality of contrast media

*Abbreviations:* CHF, congestive heart failure; CIN, contrast-induced nephropathy; NSAIDs, nonsteroidal antiinflammatory drugs.

anemia; renal transplant; and other toxins such as NSAID, cyclosporine, aminoglycosides, and furosemide. Procedure-related factors include multiple contrast media injections within 72 hours, intra-arterial injection site, high volume of contrast, and high osmolality of contrast (see **Box 1**).

Risk scores can be assigned to predetermine patients who are at increased risk (**Fig. 1**). Patients with a lower score were shown to have a mortality risk of 1.9% to 2% versus patients with a higher score who had a mortality risk of 31% to 33% (**Fig. 2**).[9]

## PROGNOSTIC IMPLICATIONS OF BASELINE RENAL INSUFFICIENCY AND CIN

Minimal change in baseline renal function may not be detected by serum creatinine measurements; however, it influences clinical outcomes. Patients with lower GFRs have an increased mortality associated with renal insufficiency, regardless of whether they develop CIN (**Fig. 3**).[10] Surgically treated patients in the BARI (Bypass Angioplasty Revascularization Investigation) trial plus registry showed a 46% mortality rate in patients with chronic kidney disease and diabetes versus a 5% mortality rate in patients without DM or renal disease.[11] In the Controlled Abciximab and Device Investigation to Lower Late Angioplasty Complications trial, 1-year survival was significantly decreased in patients with a creatinine clearance of less than 20 mL/min. The 30-day mortality was 16.2% in the CI-AKI group, with 1-year mortality of 23.3%. The patients who did not have CI-AKI had a 30-day mortality of 1.2% and 1-year mortality of 3.2%.[12] Even increase (0.25 mg/dL) in serum creatinine level increased in-hospital mortality by 4% to 30%.[13,14]

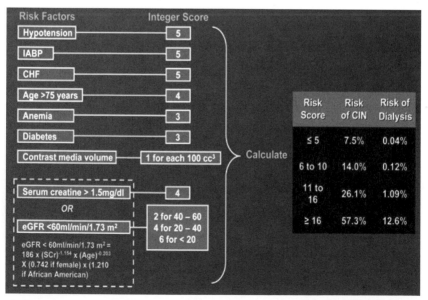

**Fig. 1.** Risk score for prediction of CIN. (*From* Mehran R, Aymong ED, Nikolsky E, et al. A simple risk score for prediction of contrast-induced nephropathy after percutaneous coronary intervention: development and initial validation. J Am Coll Cardiol 2004;4(7):1393–9; with permission.)

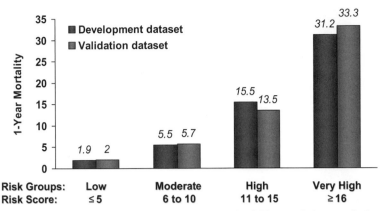

Prognostic significance of the proposed risk score for CIN extended to prediction of one-year mortality.

**Fig. 2.** CIN risk score and 1-year mortality. (*From* Mehran R, Aymong ED, Nikolsky E, et al. A simple risk score for prediction of contrast-induced nephropathy after percutaneous coronary intervention: development and initial validation. J Am Coll Cardiol 2004;4(7):1393–9; with permission.)

The development of AKI usually defined as 25% increase in serum creatinine level is associated with a 20-fold increase in mortality (**Table 3**).[14] Patients who required hemodialysis had a 50% reduction in survival at 1 year, with no difference in 1-year survival between patients requiring permanent hemodialysis and temporary hemodialysis during their hospitalization. The mortality rate was the highest within 90 days after percutaneous coronary intervention (PCI) in both groups.[10]

## THERAPIES FOR CI-AKI PREVENTION

Several studies have been conducted to determine the best strategies to prevent CI-AKI (**Box 2**). The therapies that have shown either to have no benefit or to cause harm include dopamine, mannitol, furosemide, atrial natriuretic peptide, mixed endothelin

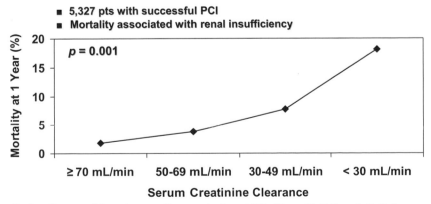

**Fig. 3.** Baseline renal function predicts survival post-PCI. (*From* McCullough P. Outcomes of contrast-induced nephropathy: experience in patients undergoing cardiovascular intervention. Catheter Cardiovasc Interv 2006;67:335; with permission.)

**Table 3**
**In-hospital mortality in patients developing CIN**

| Study | Contrast Study | Number of Patients | Incidence of CIN (%) | In-hospital Mortality (%) Control Group | CIN Group | P Value |
|---|---|---|---|---|---|---|
| Levy. JAMA 1996[15] | CT head and body: cardiac and peripheral angiography | 16,248 | 1.1 | 7 | 34 | <0.001 |
| Rihal. Circ 2002[16] | Coronary procedures (balloon angioplasty, stenting, atherecto my) | 7586 | 3.3 | 1.4 | 22 | <0.0001 |
| Bartholomew. AJC 2004[17] | Coronary interventions | 20,479 | 2 | 1 | 21 | <0.0001 |

From McCullough P. Outcomes of contrast-induced nephropathy: experience in patients undergoing cardiovascular intervention. Catheter Cardiovasc Interv 2006;67:335; with permission.

antagonists, and calcium channel blockers.[18–20] Dopamine, mannitol, and furosemide cause increase in prerenal perfusion by promoting dehydration or renal artery constriction. Calcium channel blockers have not shown to be of any benefit.

Therapies that have shown to be beneficial include infusion of sodium bicarbonate 0.9 NS, LOCM, and N-acetylcysteine.[18,21] Preventing dehydration and administration of 0.9 NS 4 to 6 hours before procedure has shown to be of some benefit. Starting sodium bicarbonate 1 hour before procedure has been shown to provide additional benefit in the higher-risk groups. Postprocedure hydration should be continued and serum creatinine reassessed in 24 to 48 hours. N-acetylcysteine 600 to 1200 mg orally 2 doses 24 hours before the procedure and the day of the procedure has shown benefit in some studies (but not all) but does not cause harm. Some believe that the creatinine level is artificially lowered without actually providing renal protection.

**Box 2**
**Prevention of CI-AKI**

*No benefit or may cause harm*

- Mannitol
- Furosemide
- Dopamine
- Calcium channel blockers
- Atrial natriuretic peptide
- Mixed endothelial antagonists
- Dopamine

*Beneficial*

LOCM

Saline

N-acetylcysteine

Sodium bicarbonate

*Data from* Refs.[9,15–17,19]

Administering LOCM prevents intrarenal injury. A meta-analysis of 39 trials that compared HOCM with LOCM showed a significant reduction in CI-AKI.[22] Patients who had diabetes and serum creatinine levels between 1.5 and 3.5 mg/dL who underwent coronary or aortofemoral angiography with LOCM contrast had a significantly less incidence of CI-AKI than the group that received HOCM contrast.[23]

## SUMMARY

The most important independent predictor of poor outcomes post-PCI is CI-AKI. It remains a frequent source of acute renal failure and is associated with increased morbidity and mortality and higher resource use. There are several factors that predispose patients to CI-AKI. Preventive measures before the procedure as well as careful postprocedure management should be routine in all patients.

Nephrotoxic drugs, such as NSAIDs and antibiotics, should be discontinued. The role of N-acetylcysteine is unclear, but administration should be considered. The infusion of sodium bicarbonate may be useful, but more definitive data are needed. The amount of contrast should be limited, and LOCM are better than HOCM. Iso-osmolar contrast agents do not seem to be superior to LOCM. Careful catheter techniques are needed to reduce clotting. These techniques include frequent flushing and avoiding back-bleeding into the guiding catheter.

### *Nursing Implications*

Patients undergoing angiography should be assessed for risk level of developing AKI secondary to contrast agents. All patients should have a preprocedure creatinine, and a GFR should be calculated. Patients should also be screened for recent radiographic contrast administration (computed tomographic scan or interventional contrast media studies), the presence of DM, or a prior history of AKI. Diuretics should be withheld the day of the procedure to prevent dehydration. NSAIDs should be discontinued, but aspirin and clopidogrel bisulfate should be administered before the procedure.

Once a patient has been identified as high risk, cardiac catherization laboratory staff should anticipate early admission for preprocedure hydration. Preprocedure areas will need to accommodate these patients because 4 to 6 hours of intravenous (IV) 0.9 NS can only be given in the hospital setting. The infusion rate and total volume of hydration should be reduced in patients with a history of CHF. Sodium bicarbonate infusion should be started 1 hour to procedure, in addition to hydration in high-risk group. Two doses of oral N-acetylcysteine 600 to 1200 mg should have been given the day before admission and 2 doses on the day of the procedure. The use of preprinted order sheets allows for individual practitioner preference and prevents the need for clarification (**Fig. 4**).

Patients need to be monitored for hemodynamic tolerance to IV hydration. Patients should be assessed for pulmonary vascular congestion before starting the infusion as well during the infusion. Symptoms of pulmonary vascular congestion include lung sounds consistent with rales, orthopnea, or hypoxia. Patients may become restless and complain of difficulty breathing. Strict intake and output are necessary to determine if the patient is adequately hydrated.

N-acetylcysteine is not very palatable, and mixing with juice or soda makes the ingestion more tolerable. Confirming that the patient had 2 doses of N-acetylcysteine the day before the procedure should be included in the preprocedure check list. If this is not possible because of lack of time due to the urgency of the case, then 2 doses postprocedure should be given.

Administration of LOCM should be used in patients who are at high risk for AKI. The amount of contrast given should be adequate to perform quality images, but repeated

**Beaumont**
William Beaumont Hospital

**Medication Order Pre Cardiac Catheterization / Elective**          Mylar Imprint

| DRUG SENSITIVITIES | PT. WEIGHT (KG) | PATIENT NAME | | ROOM NO. |
|---|---|---|---|---|

---

**DO NOT MAKE CHANGES TO PREPRINTED MEDICATION ORDERS**

**IV Hydration / Contrast Nephropathy Prophylaxis Protocol**

☐ 0.9% NaCl   OR   ☐ Dextrose 5% 0.45% NaCl

Start in left arm (preferably) as soon as patient is prepped, up to 12 hrs before procedure

1
☐ Ejection Fraction > 35% infuse at 1.5 ml/kg/hr (max = 150 ml/hr)
☐ Ejection Fraction ≤ 35% infuse at 1 ml/kg/hr (max = 100 ml/hr)
☐ Ejection Fraction is unavailable or serum creatinine > 1.5, infuse at 100 ml/hr; start 5 hrs before procedure
☐ Give a bolus _____ ml immediately before procedure
☐ Other IV fluid_____
**OR**
☐ Sodium Bicarbonate 150 mEq in 1000 ml Dextrose 5%; start 1 hour before procedure. Infuse a bolus of 0.45 mEq/kg bicarbonate for the first hour, then reduce rate to 0.15 mEq/kg/hour for 6 hours.

☐ Acetylcysteine (Mucomyst) 800 mg PO BID on day before and day of exposure to contrast; dilute in 2-4 ounces of soda pop or juice. Do not delay procedure when unable to initiate this protocol.

**Contrast Allergy Protocol**

2
☐ Prednisone 50 mg PO Q 6 hrs x 3 doses (13, 7, & 1 hr before procedure)
☐ Diphenhydramine (Benadryl) 50 mg IV push 5 minutes before procedure

**Antiplatelet Therapy**

3
☐ Aspirin 324 mg (81 mg x 4 chewable tablets) PO given before procedure
☐ Clopidogrel (Plavix) preferably 3 hrs pre-procedure
   ☐ 300 mg loading dose PO before procedure **OR**
   ☐ 600 mg PO before procedure **OR**
   ☐ 75 mg PO before procedure

4
☐ Hold long-acting thiazide diuretics 2 days before day of procedure; discontinue short-acting diuretics such as furosemide (Lasix), or bumetanide (Bumex), torsemide (Demadex) the day of procedure
☐ Hold NSAIDs e.g. Ibuprofen (Motrin), Vioxx, Celebrex, Bextra, Aleve 24 hrs before procedure
☐ Hold ACE inhibitor, ARBs on the day of procedure
☐ Hold metformin (Glucophage, Glucovance, Metaglip, Avandamet,) on day of procedure

**ATTENTION PHYSICIAN:**

– ORDER MEDICATIONS by checking the box in front of the medication and completing the blanks where necessary.

– **Use a ballpoint pen only and press firmly.**

– Indicate first time medication is needed.

– Authorization is given for dispensing by non-proprietary name under the WBH Formulary System. Any trade names shown in parenthesis are intended for medication name recognition and may not be the brand dispensed. To order a specific brand medication the standard medication order form (386) must be used.

Patients undergoing cath/possible PTCA will be given aspirin.

Patients will not be started on Plavix unless specified on the Preadmission Preprocedure form.

| Physician Signature | | | | Page No. | Date | Time |
|---|---|---|---|---|---|---|
| Noted by Unit Secretary | Date | Time | Noted by R.N. | | Date | Time |

817 SEP 04 OS7          WHITE – Medical Record  •  CANARY – Pharmacy  •  PINK – Nursing

**Fig. 4.** Analysis in-hospital morality with CIN. (*Courtesy of* William Beaumont Hospital, Royal Oak, MI; with permission.)

injections should be avoided. The total contrast volume should be closely monitored and consideration given to complexity of the intervention in patients with multivessel disease. When possible, additional contrast should be avoided when information can be obtained from noninvasive methods. For example, eliminating the left ventriculogram may be appropriate when ejection fraction is available by 2-dimensional echocardiogram.

Postprocedure monitoring should include hourly urine output in the high-risk patients. Maintaining adequate urine output (100 mL/h) may require the use of a Foley catheter for accurate measurement. Avoiding nephrotoxic medications, including aminoglycosides, amphotericin B, cisplatin/carboplatin, and NSAIDs, prevents further tubular epithelial cell damage.[24]

Hypotension should be avoided to prevent low renal perfusion. In the event of hypotension, fluid resuscitation should be used, avoiding dopamine and epinephrine.

Underlying cause of hypotension should be treated. If patient has experienced an excessive blood loss, administration of blood products may be necessary.

Renal function should be assessed 3 to 7 days after the procedure. Patients need to be counseled on the importance of having additional blood work done as an outpatient. NSAIDs and other nephrotoxic medications should be avoided. Postprocedure instructions should include this information.

## REFERENCES

1. Voel MD, Nelan MA, McDaniel MC, et al. The important properties of contrast media: focus on viscosity. J Invasive Cardiol 2007;19(3):1A–9A.
2. Grines CL, Schreiber TL, Savas V, et al. A randomized trial of low osmolar ionic versus nonionic contrast media in patients with myocardial infarction or unstable angina undergoing percutaneous transluminal coronary angioplasty. J Am Coll Cardiol 1996;27:1381–6.
3. McCullough PA, Adam A, Becker CR, et al. Risk prediction of contrast-induced nephropathy. Am J Cardiol 2006;98(Suppl S1):27–36.
4. Mehran R, Dangas G, Gruberg L, et al. The detrimental impact of chronic renal insufficiency and diabetes mellitus on late prognosis after percutaneous coronary interventions. Cardiovascular Research Foundation Washington, DC. J Am Coll Cardiol 2000;73:878–6.
5. Laskey WK, Jenkins C, Selzer F, et al. Volume-to-creatinine clearance ratio: a pharmacokinetically based risk factor for prediction of early creatinine increase after percutaneous coronary intervention. J Am Coll Cardiol 2007;50:584–90.
6. Campbell DR, Flemming BK, Mason WF, et al. A comparative study of the nephrotoxicity of iohexol, lopamidol and loxaglate in peripheral angiography. Can Assoc Radiol J 1990;41(3):133–7.
7. Nikolsky E, Mehran R, Lasic Z, et al. Low hematocrit predicts contrast-induced nephropathy after percutaneous coronary interventions. Kidney Int 2005;6:706–13.
8. Mehran R, Aymong ED, Nikolsky E, et al. A simple risk score for prediction of contrast-induced nephropathy after percutaneous coronary intervention: development and initial validation. J Am Coll Cardiol 2004;4(7):1393–9.
9. McCullough PA, Bertrand ME, Brinker JA, et al. A meta-analysis of the renal safety of isosmolar iodixanol compared to low-osmolar contrast media. J Am Coll Cardiol 2006;48(4):692–9.
10. Szczech LA, Best PJ, Crowley E, et al. Bypass Angioplasty Revascularization Investigation (BARI) Investigators. Outcomes of patients with chronic renal insufficiency in the bypass angioplasty revascularization investigation. Circulation 2002;105:2253–8.
11. Sadeghi HM, Stone GW, Grines CL, et al. Impact of renal insufficiency in patients undergoing primary angioplasty for acute myocardial infarction. Circulation 2003; 108:2769–75.
12. Weishord SD, Chen H, Stone RA, et al. Associations of increases in serum creatinine with mortality and length of hospital stay after coronary angiography. J Am Soc Nephrol 2006;10:2871–7.
13. Gruberg L, Mintz GS, Mehran R, et al. The prognostic implications of further renal function deteriorating within 48 hours of interventional coronary procedures in patients with pre-existent chronic renal insufficiency. J Am Coll Cardiol 2000;36:1542–8.
14. Gruberg L, Curry B, Duncan CC, et al. Does contemporary percutaneous coronary intervention improve the otherwise dismal prognosis of patients with end stage renal disease on dialysis? Circulation 1999;100(Suppl I):I-366.

15. Levy EM, Viscoli CM, Horwitz RI. The effect of acute renal failure on mortality. A cohort analysis. JAMA 1996;275:1489–94.
16. Rihal CS, Textor SC, Grill DE, et al. Incidence and prognostic importance of acute renal failure after percutaneous coronary intervention. Circulation 2002;105: 2259–64.
17. Bartholomew BA, Harjai KJ, Dukkipati S. Impact of nephropathy after percutaneous coronary intervention and a method for risk stratification. Am J Cardiol 2004;93:1515–19.
18. Weisberg LS, Kurnik BR. Risk of radiocontrast nephropathy in patients with and without diabetes mellitus. Kidney Int 1994;45(1):259–65.
19. Solomon R, Werener C, Mann D, et al. Effects of saline, mannitol, and furosemide to prevent acute decreases in renal function induced by radiocontrast agents. N Engl J Med 1994;331(21):1416–20.
20. Wang A, Bashore T, Holcslaw T, et al. Randomized prospective double-blind multicenter trial of an endothelin receptor antagonist in the prevention of contrast nephrotoxicity [abstract]. J Am Soc Nephrol 1998;9:137.
21. Carraro M, Mancini W, Artero M, et al. Dose effect of nitrendipine on urinary enzymes and microproteins following non-ionic radiocontrast administration. Nephrol Dial Transplant 1996;11(3):444–8.
22. Barrett BJ, Carlisle EJ. Meta-analysis of the relative nephrotoxicity of high- and low-osmolality iodinated contrast media. Radiology 1993;188(1):171–8.
23. Mehran R. Contrast induced nephropathy remains a serious complication of PCI. J Interv Cardiol 2007;20:236–40.
24. Taber SS, Mueller BA. Drug-Associated renal dysfunction. Crit Care Clin 2006;22: 357–74.

# Treatment Options for Superficial Venous Insufficiency

Gail Egan Sansivero, MS, ANP[a,b,*]

KEYWORDS

• Varicose veins • Thermal ablation • Sclerotherapy
• Phlebectomy

Chronic venous insufficiency is a disease that has been documented for more than 2000 years. Hippocrates noted its presence and attempted to induce thrombosis with iron to reduce patients' symptoms. Other middle age physicians resorted to bloodletting to alleviate discomfort. Although the first attempts of ligation and stripping of varicose veins were carried out in AD 660, it was not until the introduction of local and general anesthesia that definitive vein treatment became more common and more effective.

Today, there are many more treatment options available for patients with chronic venous insufficiency, many of which are substantially less invasive than those offered even 10 or 20 years ago. This article describes the treatment options that are available today for chronic venous insufficiency, along with nursing care before and after treatment.

Chronic venous insufficiency is caused by venous reflux, or the backward flow of blood in the venous system. When venous valves are incompetent, blood is allowed to flow backward, resulting in venous hypertension, distention, and bulging of lower extremity veins. Varicose veins are superficial veins of the lower extremities, which have become abnormally dilated, twisted, and elongated because of venous insufficiency (**Fig. 1**). Symptoms are typically magnified in distal portions of the legs where gravity exerts its most profound effects. Varicose veins is a common venous disease estimated to affect more than 25 million adults in the United States and as many as 20% to 40% of adults in the Western world.[1] Approximately 2% of the health care budget is spent on the treatment of chronic venous disease.[2]

The author has a consulting relationship with AngioDynamics Inc.
[a] Interventional Radiology, Community Care Physicians, 43 New Scotland Avenue, MC-113, Albany, NY 12208, USA
[b] Department of Radiology, Albany Medical College, MC-113, 47 New Scotland Avenue, Albany, NY 12208, USA
* Corresponding author. Department of Radiology, Albany Medical College, MC-113, 47 New Scotland Avenue, Albany, NY 12208.
E-mail address: sansivg@mail.amc.edu

Perioperative Nursing Clinics 5 (2010) 111–124
doi:10.1016/j.cpen.2010.02.005
1556-7931/10/$ – see front matter © 2010 Published by Elsevier Inc.

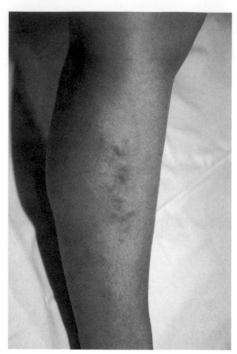

**Fig. 1.** Typical appearance of prominent superficial veins in a patient with chronic venous insufficiency. These veins are called varicose veins. Note the hyperpigmentation.

Chronic venous insufficiency is more likely to occur in women, the elderly, and those with a family history of venous disease. In more severe cases, venous insufficiency can be disabling, causing difficulty with walking and standing. Unfortunately, many patients do not seek treatment because they may think that treatment options are limited or that their problem is strictly cosmetic and thus not worthy of further investigation.

## ANATOMY AND PATHOPHYSIOLOGY

The venous system of the lower extremities can be divided into the deep system (femoral, popliteal, and crural veins) and the superficial system (great and short saphenous veins). Perforator veins connect the systems, generally allowing one-way flow from the superficial to the deep system. The systems join at the saphenofemoral junction (SFJ) in the groin area and at the saphenopopliteal junction behind the knee. Reticular veins are smaller veins that come off the superficial system and that are often easily visible through the skin. Telangiectasias, or spider veins, are small caliber vessels that often have a web-like appearance. Telangiectasias are the most superficial of varicose veins, and are often seen in the lateral thigh, medial and lateral knee, and ankle (**Fig. 2**).

## INCIDENCE AND RISK FACTORS

Superficial venous incompetence is a common disorder, affecting up to 25% of women and 15% of men with varicose veins.[2] In up to 75% of patients, great saphenous vein (GSV) reflux is the underlying cause. Other risk factors for the development

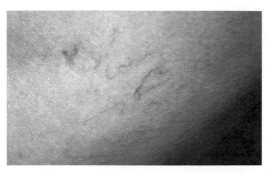

**Fig. 2.** Typical appearance of very superficial, small caliber but dilated veins known as telangiectasias or spider veins.

of chronic venous insufficiency include pregnancy, estrogen therapy, obesity, family history, phlebitis, and previous leg injury. Risk for development of varicose veins increases with age, with the risk tripling in those older than 35 years.[3] It is estimated that varicose veins affect 50% of the US population by the age of 50 years and 75% of women by the age of 70 years.[4] Certain genetic disorders, particularly Klippel-Trénaunay syndrome, may predispose the patient to the development of varicose veins, most likely because of impairment of the venous muscle pump function and valvular incompetence. Further studies of the genetic origin of chronic venous insufficiency are warranted. There may also be environmental risk factors such as prolonged sitting or standing. Despite the extent of venous disease in the adult population, the exact mechanism and determinants of varicose vein formation are still unknown. Theories propose that there may be primary changes in the structure of valves, or that inflammation may play a role.[1]

## PRESENTATION AND ASSESSMENT

Patients present with a spectrum of symptoms depending on the severity of their disease and their activity level. Some patients who have telangiectasia alone may be asymptomatic. These patients often present for evaluation for cosmetic reasons, being dissatisfied with the appearance of prominent veins on the lower extremities. They may be particularly unhappy with their appearance in warmer weather, when clothing choices may make their varicosities more visible.

Patients with large varicosities often report feelings of pain, burning, and/or fatigue in the legs. Patients may report that their legs feel heavy or warm or that they have itching or tingling at the site of prominent veins. Symptoms are typically worsened at the end of the day (after standing/walking) and in warmer weather. If a varicosity is in the posterior lower extremity, patients may complain that discomfort is increased when additional pressure is applied to the site by sitting in a chair or car. Edema may be present and often worsens during the course of the day after periods of standing, ambulation, and exercise.

In some cases, patients may seek treatment for abrupt onset of pain and warmth in a focal area. There may be a tender, palpable cordlike area just beneath the skin, which generally represents superficial thrombophlebitis. Although diagnosis can generally be made clinically, ultrasonography is warranted to rule out deep venous disease. Untreated superficial thrombophlebitis may result in lipodermatosclerosis and venous ulceration. Symptomatic treatment with nonsteroidal antiinflammatory drugs (NSAIDs), elevation, and moist heat is often effective.

In severe cases, there may be extensive edema, severe telangiectasia formation, skin discoloration, and/or venous ulceration.

## CLINICAL EVALUATION
### History

Patients should be asked about any family history of varicose veins, particularly in siblings and parents. The patient's personal history should also include

Age at onset and duration of symptoms.
Effect of pregnancy (if applicable) on symptoms.
Character, severity, and location of symptoms.
Effect of symptoms on lifestyle.
Measures that improve or worsen symptoms.
Any previous vein therapy.
Previous or concurrent use of compression stockings.
History of any clotting disorders, deep vein thrombosis, pulmonary embolism, or hypercoagulable state.

## PHYSICAL EXAMINATION

Physical examination, including ultrasound evaluation, should be performed with the patient in a standing position. The legs should be examined for overall color and temperature, symmetry, muscle tone, capillary refill, arterial pulses, edema, location and diameter of varicosities, presence of venous malformations, telangiectasia, or skin discoloration caused by scarring, ulcers, or venous stasis. The patient should be asked to identify the areas that are most symptomatic. The patient should also be specifically asked about the presence of any symptoms of pelvic pressure, labial varicosities, and dyspareunia, because these conditions may indicate that there are varicosities in the pelvis, known as pelvic congestion syndrome.

Ultrasonography using color flow duplex imaging is the gold standard for noninvasive anatomic and functional assessment of venous reflux. A high-frequency linear array transducer of 7.5 to 13 MHz is appropriate for most lower extremity imaging. The Doppler ultrasonography uses directional flow detection to localize venous valvular incompetence. The duplex combines echo pulsing with Doppler velocity recording using mechanical or pneumatic stimuli. This feature allows direct visualization of veins and identifies blood flow through valves.

The patient is examined in the standing position. Imaging begins at the groin with the identification of the SFJ and extends to the ankle. Venous reflux is initiated by imaging the vein while the patient performs the Valsalva maneuver or while direct manual compression is applied to the calf. Pneumatic cuff compression may also be used to initiate reflux, particularly if the examining clinician is working alone. Venous reflux is identified if retrograde flow is noted and lasts for more than 0.5 seconds.

Using duplex imaging, the clinician is able to identify the exact location of venous reflux, as well as the location and size of varicose and perforator vessels. Data to be determined from the duplex ultrasonography are[5]

- The saphenous junctions that are incompetent, their locations and diameters.
- The extent of reflux in the saphenous veins of the thighs and legs and the diameter of these saphenous veins. The number, location, and diameter and function of the incompetent perforating vessels.
- Other relevant veins that show reflux.

- The source of filling of all superficial varices, if not from the veins already described.
- Veins that are hypoplastic, atretic, absent, or have been removed.
- The state of the deep venous system, including competence of valves and evidence of previous venous thrombosis.

## CLASSIFICATION OF VENOUS DISEASE

Venous disease of the lower extremities is classified according to the severity, cause, site, and specific abnormality using the CEAP classification.[6] The CEAP system was developed by an international ad hoc committee of the American Venous Forum to develop consistent nomenclature for describing venous diseases.[6] The elements of the classification system are

Clinical severity,
Etiology or cause,
Anatomy, and
Pathophysiology.

Clinical severity is easily observed and can be classified without special tests.

| Grade | Description |
|-------|-------------|
| C 0 | No evidence of venous disease |
| C 1 | Superficial spider veins (reticular veins) only |
| C 2 | Simple varicose veins only |
| C 3 | Varicose veins and edema |
| C 4 | Varicose veins and evidence of venous stasis skin changes |
| C 5 | Varicose veins and a healed venous ulceration |
| C 6 | Varicose veins and an open venous ulceration |

## TREATMENT OPTIONS
### Conservative Therapy

Compression stockings are an important component of chronic venous disease treatment. Compression stockings are available in different classes or strengths, which is measured in millimeters of mercury, with a higher number referring to a stocking that exerts more compression. The stockings are designed with a gradient, with the tightest portion of the stocking in the foot area. Compression stockings act by augmenting the pumping action of the calf muscles to return blood to the heart. As such, compression stockings may ameliorate symptoms and reduce edema. The beneficial effects of compression stockings are directly related to the time that they are worn, and their benefits quickly dissipate when use is discontinued. Stockings should be applied as soon as the patient arises in the morning, when edema will be minimal, and should be worn throughout the day. Because the legs are elevated at night, the stockings need not be worn during sleeping hours. Patients who are not candidates for further intervention may require life-long compression stocking use.

For patients with chronic venous insufficiency who are candidates for thermal ablation, a stocking with compression of 30 to 40 mm Hg is generally prescribed. This stocking compares to a stocking with compression less than 20 mm Hg, which is useful for prevention of deep vein thrombosis in the perioperative period.[7] Compression stockings should extend to the groin for adequate compression along the course of the incompetent vein. Stockings are available in many styles, including thigh high, chap style (thigh high with an attached waistband), and pantyhose. For patients with disease confined below the knee, knee-high stockings are adequate. Careful measurement of the patient's lower extremities (circumference and length) is necessary to ensure an appropriate fit. Custom stockings may be necessary in some patients.

There is a lack of consensus regarding the optimal stocking strength needed for treatment before and after other interventions, as well as the duration of use after invasive procedures. The patient's ability to successfully don a stocking should be considered before prescription. Patients who are obese, who have balance difficulties, or who have severe arthritis may have significant difficulty in putting on their stockings.

## Minimally Invasive Treatment Options

Endovenous thermal ablation by either laser or radiofrequency (RF) ablation has emerged as an effective alternative to surgical stripping in many patients with chronic venous insufficiency. These minimally invasive options have shown high clinical efficacy with venous occlusions and symptomatic improvements while maintaining a low complication profile. Clinical success rates of greater than 90% have been reported for thermal ablation techniques.[8,9] The success of any thermal ablation technique depends on elimination of the highest point of deep to superficial incompetence. That is, the entire segment of incompetent vein must be treated.

RF ablation uses electromagnetic radiation in the frequency range of 3 kHz to 300 GHz. This high-frequency current is used to generate heat, which in turn causes denaturation of collagen when in contact with the vein wall. This denaturation results in irreversible shrinkage of collagen and thus of the vessel wall. RF systems consist of collapsible electrodes that are introduced intraluminally. The catheter tip is navigated to the SFJ, and the catheter is slowly withdrawn at 85°C.

In a study of 194 patients with 252 treated GSV abnormalities, Proebstle and colleagues[10] noted immediate vein occlusion after segmental thermal ablation in 100% of patients, with significant relief from symptoms as early as 3 days postprocedure. Edema and pain were reduced in all subjects. Complications included paresthesias (3.2%) and superficial thrombophlebitis (0.8%). Other minor complications included hematoma, skin hyperpigmentation, and erythema.

Several trials have compared RF ablation with vein stripping. The largest, the EVOLVeS trial, was a multicenter randomized trial that compared quality-of-life factors. All patients in the trial who were treated with RF reported significantly less postprocedure pain, fewer adverse events, and faster recovery. At 2 years posttreatment, comparable results for vein closure (91.2% for RF ablation, 91.7% for stripping) were obtained.[11]

Endovenous laser ablation (EVLA) uses a laser as a heat source. The term laser is an acronym for light amplification by stimulated emission of radiation. Medical lasers are available in a variety of wavelengths. All lasers use light from the visible and infrared portions of the optical electromagnetic spectrum. EVLA can be used to abolish reflux by inducing thermal injury to the venous endothelium, leading to fibrous sclerosis of the treated vein.

In a series of 60 consecutive EVLAs, Kim and Paxton[8] reported initial treatment success rates of 94.7%. The investigators noted that a larger saphenous vein diameter was associated with early treatment failures in 3 patients.

Theivacumar and colleagues[12] evaluated 582 patients at 6 and 12 weeks after EVLA for closure in 644 treated sites. The investigators defined success as presence of noncompressible vein or absence of the treated vein along with the absence of color flow duplex ultrasonography while maintaining competence of the SFJ. The length of the treated vein and the vein diameter did not influence outcome. Vein diameter was significantly reduced at the time of treatment because of catheter-induced spasm with cannulation and the addition of tumescent anesthetic.

Not all patients are candidates for surgical or minimally invasive vein treatment. Patients with an allergy to local anesthetics and who have DVT or a history of DVT with incomplete recanalization or active superficial thrombophlebitis are best treated with conservative therapy using compression.[13]

Vuylsteke and colleagues[14] compared the efficacy of EVLA with that of surgical stripping in 164 patients with varicose veins caused by GSV reflux. Postoperative morbidity, use of analgesics, and time spent away from work were recorded. Minor postoperative complications were common in both groups and included saphenous nerve paresthesia, hematoma, and ecchymoses. Patients treated with EVLA reported significantly less postprocedure pain, and used substantially fewer sick days (18.9 days for the stripping group, 4.1 days for the EVLA group). The procedural cost for EVLA, however, may be slightly higher because of the costs associated with the catheter and laser.

Few comparisons between RF ablation of the GSV and endovenous laser therapy have been reported. In a series of 92 patients with 130 treated limbs, Puggioni and colleagues[15] compared the thermal ablation techniques in terms of efficacy and complication profile. GSV occlusion was achieved in more than 90% of cases in both groups at 1-month postprocedure follow-up evaluation. Complications included thrombus protrusion into the common femoral vein, superficial thrombophlebitis, edema, and excessive pain.

## PROCEDURE
### Patient Preparation

Oral foods and fluids need not be withheld from patients for these procedures, which are typically performed using only local or tumescent anesthesia. In some cases, small doses of opioids such as hydrocodone/acetaminophen or benzodiazepines may be given just before the procedure. In anxious or sensitive patients, these medications may make the administration of local anesthetic more tolerable.

Patients are not required to discontinue use of antiplatelet agents, aspirin products, or anticoagulants before the procedure. Patients who routinely take other medications such as antihypertensives should take them on the day of the procedure.

All patients should arrive in the office with a plan for transport home. Whether medicated or not, the presence of extensive local anesthetic in a limb makes driving on the treatment day impossible.

## PROCEDURE

Regardless of the type of thermal ablation selected, these procedures can be performed in an outpatient setting. A standard examining-room table can be used. Because the patient may be in the same position for up to an hour (including preparation time and postprocedure care), care should be taken to assure the patient's comfort with appropriate pillows and linens. The patient is positioned supine, often with the leg to be treated elevated to reduce blood volume in the target vein. The limb is prepared with a standard solution of chlorhexidine or similar solution. The point of access is confirmed with ultrasonography, and a small volume of local anesthetic is administered. The saphenous vein is accessed with a small-gauge (21-gauge) needle (**Fig. 3**), after which a small guidewire (0.018 in) is advanced approximately 20 cm. A small dermatotomy is made in the skin to allow a sheath to be placed once the introducer needle has been withdrawn. This sheath is advanced to the SFJ, which is identified on simultaneous ultrasonography. Before application of thermal energy, tumescent anesthesia is administered.

Tumescent anesthesia is a technique that allows delivery of diluted local anesthetic to the skin and soft tissue. Regional subcutaneous infiltration of a large volume of diluted lidocaine mixed with epinephrine causes the targeted tissue to become swollen and firm (tumescent) and permits the procedure to be performed with minimal amounts of other systemic medications, if needed. The tumescent anesthetic is administered under ultrasound guidance, with the solution directed into the fascial space surrounding the vein (**Fig. 4**). The anesthetic provides pain control during the application of thermal energy, helps constrict the vein around the catheter, and serves as a heat sink or insulating barrier between the vein to be treated and the surrounding soft tissues. Administration can be facilitated by use of an infusion pump, which delivers the solution at a predetermined rate and is controlled by a foot pedal. A typical mixture of tumescent anesthesia is normal saline, 200 mL, mixed with 1% lidocaine with epinephrine, 30 mL, and 10 mL sodium bicarbonate.

Once the tumescent anesthetic administration is complete, the RF probe or laser fiber is passed through the sheath (**Fig. 5**), such that it protrudes just beyond the tip of the sheath. The system is then activated, with heat applied to the saphenous vein while the system is slowly retracted until it is withdrawn from the initial puncture site (**Fig. 6**). Although the entire procedure may take up to 45 minutes, the application of thermal energy takes only a few minutes.

## POST-TREATMENT CARE

Upon removal of the sheath, hemostasis is generally quickly achieved. The operator may compress the treated vein to remove any residual blood. Because only a small dermatotomy has been made, there is no need to suture the site. A small skin closure device may be used, although many clinicians simply apply a dry sterile dressing. A compression stocking is then immediately applied (**Fig. 7**). The stocking is left on for 24 hours and then worn for 2 to 4 weeks while the patient is awake.

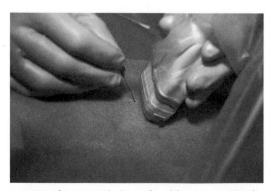

**Fig. 3.** Access to the great saphenous vein is made with a 21-gauge microintroducer needle. The needle is guided into the target vein using ultrasonography.

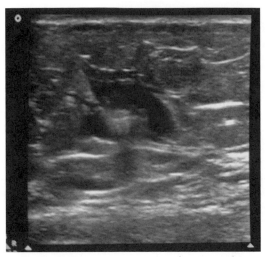

**Fig. 4.** Tumescent anesthetic administered around the GSV. Note the appearance of the sheath within the vein, the vein wall, and the surrounding anesthetic, which appears the darkest.

Patients are encouraged to resume their normal activities, including walking, immediately. The patient may take a shower 24 hours after treatment. Activities that would substantially dilate the lower extremity vessels, such as immersion in hot tubs, vigorous aerobic exercise, and hot showers or baths, should be avoided until the patient is seen in follow-up, usually within a month.

The treated limb is somewhat uncomfortable for up to 2 weeks after treatment. Patients may describe a pulling or hard rope sensation in the inner thigh area, which is typically worse in the groin. The patients are also likely to notice a lumpy sensation along the course of the treated vein, which is related to the administration of large

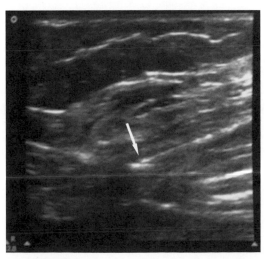

**Fig. 5.** The laser fiber is advanced into the venous sheath. Only the tip of the laser fiber emits heat (*arrow*).

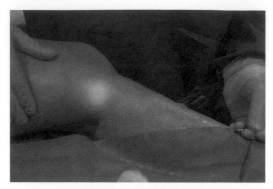

**Fig. 6.** The laser fiber is slowly withdrawn in a retrograde fashion over a period of 1 to 4 minutes, depending on the length of the vein to be treated. The vein may be compressed manually as the laser fiber and sheath are retracted. Note the glow of the laser under the patient's skin.

volumes of tumescent anesthetic. Ecchymoses are common and resolve within a week or so. Discomfort is typically well managed with over-the-counter nonsteroidal antiinflammatory medications.

Patients should be clearly advised in immediately reportable conditions, which include shortness of breath, chest pain, uncontrolled pain, increasing lower extremity edema, and excessive erythema or heat at the site.

### Phlebectomy

Many patients require follow-up treatment after thermal ablation therapy to treat smaller, residual varicosities. Treatment options include ambulatory phlebectomy and sclerotherapy.

Ambulatory microphlebectomy is used for removal of large, superficial, and tortuous varicosities through the use of hooks and clamps. This procedure can be performed concomitantly with thermal ablation or during follow-up.[16] After preparation of the leg and administration of local anesthetic, a needle (18 gauge) or small blade (number 11) is used to make 1- to 2-mm incisions. These incisions should be made parallel to the long axis of the leg whereby the normal skin lines are followed. A small hook is inserted into the incision and used to grab the vein and pull it through the incision. As the vein is removed, it is grasped with a forcep and gently pulled. These steps are repeated along the course of the vein.

Fernandez and colleagues[17] reported on 1652 patients treated with EVLA and microphlebectomy in the same treatment session. The investigators noted that

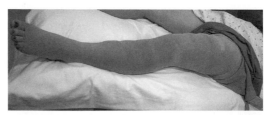

**Fig. 7.** A small dry sterile dressing is applied to the puncture site, and the entire extremity is covered with a compression stocking immediately on completion of the vein ablation procedure.

although GSV reflux is the most common underlying cause for varicose veins, patients often have other sources of superficial reflux, including the short saphenous vein. By treating all sources of the patient's reflux, Fernandez and colleagues[17] aimed to reduce intervention to 1 treatment visit. No statistically significant differences were noted in postprocedure pain scores in patients treated with EVLA and microphlebectomy as compared with patients treated with EVLA alone.

Patient preparation and postprocedure care are same as for the thermal ablation techniques. Most patients tolerate phlebectomy extremely well. The most common complication after phlebectomy is hematoma formation. Careful attention to accurate application of the postprocedure dressing and compression helps minimize this risk. Significant complications such as infection are rare.

## Sclerotherapy

Sclerotherapy is designed to obliterate small incompetent veins. A sclerosing agent is one that causes inflammation and scarring of the vein's endothelium, resulting in closure of the vein. The only Food and Drug Administration–approved sclerosant in the United States is sodium tetradecyl sulfate (Sotradecol). After skin preparation, the veins are accessed with a small (30-gauge) needle attached to a 1- to 3-mL syringe containing the sclerosing agent. Aspiration for blood return is obtained, and after confirmation of accurate needle tip placement, the sclerosant is injected. The sclerosant irreversibly damages the vein endothelium, causing it to scar down. Sclerotherapy can be used for reticular and spider veins, although the small diameter of spider veins precludes a blood return on access.

Access into the target vein can be enhanced with the use of transilluminating devices. These devices are typically engineered in a ring fashion, with the light source contained within the ring. The light illuminates the surface underneath the skin, which allows improved visualization of spider and reticular veins. These transilluminating systems can also be used during initial patient consultation to help identify veins and pathways.

Ultrasound-guided foam sclerotherapy may be used to maximize the effect of the sclerosing agent. The sclerosing agent is agitated with air to form a foamlike solution, which is injected and then tracked with ultrasonography. Using a foamlike solution increases the surface area of the drug. As such, the drug displaces rather than

---

**Box 1**
**Instructions before your vein treatment procedure**

You are scheduled to undergo a vein treatment procedure to treat your varicose veins. This procedure should take approximately 1 hour and will be performed in the physician's office. Please follow the following simple instructions in getting ready for your procedure:

1. We have prescribed the following mild sedative:————————————————

   Please take it ——— hour before your scheduled endovenous laser procedure.

2. You must have a friend drive you to and from your appointment. Although the laser procedure will not impair your ability to walk, the administration of local sedative and wrapping of your leg makes it best not to drive immediately after the procedure.

   Please remember to bring the following compression stockings with you:————————————————————————————————

   If you have any questions, please call our office at:

dilutes the blood, causing maximal sclerosing action. Care must be taken to carefully monitor the injection and pathway of foam sclerotherapy to reduce the risk of foam or particulate migration to the right heart and subsequent embolization to the central nervous system when a right-to-left cardiac shunt is present. Several methods to reduce this risk have been described in the literature, including elevation of the leg during treatment, compression of the SFJ, and balloon occlusion. In a study of 58 patients treated with foam sclerotherapy, Hill and colleagues[18] compared elevation, compression of the SFJ and elevation, and compression alone while the patient's right atrium and ventricle were continuously monitored with ultrasonography. Echogenic phenomena were common in patients after foam sclerotherapy, but leg elevation alone was effective in reducing target vein diameter, permitting smaller doses of sclerosant to be administered. Because foam is lighter than blood, leg elevation facilitates the persistence of foam in the treated vein and helps protect against migration to the heart.

Hyperpigmentation is the most common complication of sclerotherapy and is seen in 10% to 20% of patients. The complication typically resolves without treatment but may take 6 to 12 months to do so. Venous ulceration may occur if the sclerosant is injected subcutaneously or intra-arterially. Care should be taken to avoid extravasation.

Compression stockings are applied upon completion of sclerotherapy to prevent reflux and to reduce the diameter of the treated veins. Kern and colleagues[19] showed that patients who wore compression stockings after sclerotherapy had reduced extent of microthrombi, venous matting, and hyperpigmentation as compared with patients who did not wear compression hose after sclerotherapy.

---

**Box 2**
**Leg care after your vein treatment procedure**

Now that your procedure is complete, you may resume normal activities with only a few exceptions and suggestions:

1. You are encouraged to walk for at least 20 minutes every several hours during the day. Walking will help the leg's recovery process.

2. Please refrain from swimming, using a hot tub, or taking a hot bath for 72 hours after your procedure. You may shower and clean the treated leg, but try to avoid submerging the leg in water.

3. Please also refrain from running or vigorous exercises at the gymnasium for 2 weeks after your procedure.

4. Avoid exposure to excessive sun during the 2 weeks after the procedure.

5. It is normal to experience bruising, soreness, and a tightening sensation in the 2- to 3-week period after treatment, but these conditions should begin to subside after 2 weeks. You can take over-the-counter pain medications, such as acetaminophen (Tylenol) or ibuprofen (Advil), as needed for your discomfort.

6. You will need to wear your compression stockings for the first 24 hours after your procedure and then for the next —— days, taking them off to shower, but leaving them on for the rest of the day and night.

7. You may take your dressing off in 24 hours. If you have adhesive strips on at the site, leave them in place. They will start to dry and curl in a week or two and then can be removed.

8. If you experience bleeding or substantial pain, give us a call at:

Because local anesthetic is not typically used for sclerotherapy, patients may drive themselves to and from the procedure without limitations.

## SUMMARY

Minimally invasive treatment options have revolutionized the care of patients with chronic venous insufficiency. These techniques offer patients an outpatient-based treatment option with an acceptable morbidity profile and rapid recovery as compared with invasive methods. Further study is needed to compare the long-term outcomes of the treatment options and to further refine combination treatment strategies.

Proactive nursing care, which includes extensive patient and family education, is integral to the successful use of these technologies in the outpatient setting. Patients should be given written instructions on their initial consultation visit (**Box 1**) and again on the day of treatment (**Box 2**). Whereas most patients do quite well with only over-the-counter NSAIDs for postprocedure pain management, selected patients may require additional medication for discomfort and should be assessed as needed in the immediate postprocedure period. Although complications are generally minor and easily managed, any unusual symptoms should be evaluated immediately.

## ACKNOWLEDGMENTS

The author wishes to thank Rachelle Stepnowski, Dr Ken Mandato, and Mike Ciarmiello for their assistance with the article.

## REFERENCES

1. Raffetto JD, Khalil RA. Mechanisms of varicose vein formation: valve dysfunction and wall dilation. Phlebology 2007,23.85–98.
2. Callam JM. Epidemiology of varicose veins. Br J Surg 1994;81:167–73.
3. Sharp B, Davies AH. New concepts in the aetiology of varicose veins. Phlebology 2005;20:157–8.
4. Naom JJ, Hunter GC. Pathogenesis of varicose veins and implications for clinical management. Vascular 2007;15:242–9.
5. Coleridge-Smith P, Labropoulos N, Partsch H, et al. Duplex ultrasound investigation of the veins in chronic venous disease of the lower limbs-UIP consensus document. Part 1: basic principles. Eur J Vasc Endovasc Surg 2006;31:83–92.
6. Porter JM, Moneta GL. Reporting standards in venous disease: an update. International Consensus Committee on Chronic Venous Disease. J Vasc Surg 1995; 21:635–45.
7. Partsch H. Do we still need compression bandages? Haemodynamic effects of compression stockings and bandages. Phlebology 2006;21:132–8.
8. Kim HS, Paxton BE. Endovenous laser ablation of the great saphenous vein with a 980-nm diode laser in continuous mode: early treatment failures and successful repeat treatments. J Vasc Interv Radiol 2006;17:1449–55.
9. Mundy L, Merlin TL, Fittridge RA, et al. Systematic review of endovenous laser treatment for varicose veins. Br J Surg 2005;92:1189–94.
10. Proebstle TM, Vago B, Alm J, et al. Treatment of the incompetent great saphenous vein by endovenous radiofrequency powered segmental thermal ablation: first clinical experience. J Vasc Surg 2008;47:151–6.
11. Lurie F, Creton D, Eklof B, et al. Prospective randomized study of endovenous radiofrequency obliteration (closure procedure) versus ligation and stripping in a selected patient population (EVOLVeS Study). J Vasc Surg 2003;38:207–14.

12. Theivacumar NS, Dellagrammaticas D, Beale RJ, et al. Factors influencing the effectiveness of endovenous laser ablation (EVLA) in the treatment of great saphenous vein reflux. Eur J Vasc Endovasc Surg 2008;35:119–23.
13. Almeida JI. RFA versus laser ablation of the saphenous vein. Endovasc Today 2004;(Suppl):15–9.
14. Vuylsteke M, Van den Bussche D, Audenaert EA, et al. Endovenous laser obliteration for the treatment of primary varicose veins. Phlebology 2006;21:80–7.
15. Puggioni A, Kalra M, Carmo M, et al. Endovenous laser therapy and radiofrequency ablation of the great saphenous vein: analysis of early efficacy and complications. J Vasc Surg 2005;42:488–93.
16. Jung IM, Min SI, Heo SC, et al. Combined endovenous laser treatment and ambulatory phlebectomy for the treatment of saphenous vein incompetence. Phlebology 2008;23:172–7.
17. Fernandez CF, Roizental M, Carvallo J. Combined endovenous laser therapy and microphlebectomy in the treatment of varicose veins: efficacy and complications of a large single-center experience. J Vasc Surg 2008;48:947–52.
18. Hill D, Hamilton R, Fung T. Assessment of techniques to reduce sclerosant foam migration during ultrasound-guided sclerotherapy of the great saphenous vein. J Vasc Surg 2008;48:934–9.
19. Kern P, Ramelet AA, Wurscher R, et al. Compression after sclerotherapy for telangiectasias and reticular leg veins: a randomized controlled study. J Vasc Surg 2007;45:1212–6.

# Radiation Exposure in the Perioperative Environment

Richard J. Vetter, PhD[a,b],*

**KEYWORDS**
- Radiation • Radiation safety • Radiation protection
- Occupational radiation exposure • Radiation dose

Radiation serves an important role in the diagnosis and treatment of various medical conditions and diseases. It is a particularly important tool in the perioperative environment, in which diagnostic radiograph machines, diagnostic radiopharmaceuticals, therapeutic radiopharmaceuticals, and sealed radiation sources are used in the diagnosis, treatment, and management of many conditions and diseases. Consequently, some health care personnel in the perioperative environment are exposed to ionizing radiation in the course of their work. Essentially all of this radiation exposure is external, but there is a small possibility of internal exposure when caring for patients receiving therapeutic nuclear medicine who may contaminate their surroundings. Therefore, radiation safety practices in the perioperative environment need to take into account the potential for external and internal radiation exposure.

Early, enthusiastic medical use of radiographs and radioactive materials shortly after their discovery resulted in several deleterious biologic effects. The first accounts were published just 3 months after the discovery of x-rays was reported.[1] Risks from exposure to radiation in today's perioperative environment are small and cannot be estimated solely from epidemiologic studies of medical workers. Thus, estimates of risks to health resulting from exposure to radiation in the medical environment have been obtained primarily from other populations such as the Japanese survivors of the atomic bombings in 1945 and from patients exposed to high doses of radiation for medical purposes.[2] Some risk estimates have been obtained from studies of occupational exposure to ionizing radiation including medical workers who receive large occupational doses such as radiographers and radiologists.[3] The link between radiation exposure and excess leukemia in radiologists was reported in 1944, a year before the atomic bombings in Japan.[4] Yoshinaga and colleagues[5] recently concluded that

[a] Division of Preventive, Occupational and Aerospace Medicine, Mayo Clinic, Rochester, MN, USA
[b] Radiation Safety Office, Mayo Clinic, 200 first Street Southwest, Rochester, MN 55905, USA
* Corresponding author. Radiation Safety Office, Mayo Clinic, 200 first Street Southwest, Rochester, MN 55905.
*E-mail address:* rvetter@mayo.edu

Perioperative Nursing Clinics 5 (2010) 125–135
doi:10.1016/j.cpen.2010.02.004
1556-7931/10/$ – see front matter © 2010 Elsevier Inc. All rights reserved.

periopnursing.theclinics.com

the protracted exposure to radiation during the working lifetime of medical workers does increase their risk of leukemia. The purpose of this article is to provide a perspective of the health risks from exposure to various sources of radiation in the perioperative environment and to discuss methods for minimizing those risks.

## HEALTH EFFECTS FROM RADIATION EXPOSURE

Radiation-induced health effects from occupational exposure to radiation can be grouped into 2 general categories: deterministic effects and stochastic effects.[2,3,6] A deterministic effect is a somatic effect that increases in severity with increased radiation dose greater than a threshold dose. Deterministic effects of radiation occur only after large doses. Examples are erythema (reddening of the skin), which may occur within hours or days after exposure to a large dose of radiation, and lens opacification, which may occur years after exposure to multiple doses of radiation. A stochastic effect of radiation is one in which the probability of occurrence increases with increased exposure to radiation although the severity of the effect is independent of the radiation dose (eg, cancer). In the modern medical environment occupational radiation exposure is unlikely to result in deterministic effects if proper protection and safeguards are used. However, recent concern about cataract development has been expressed, suggesting that the threshold for cataract development may be lower than previously believed.[7] Thus, the primary concern is the risk of stochastic effects (ie, cancer and leukemia).

## RADIATION DOSE

When workers are exposed to x- and $\gamma$-radiation, some of the radiation passes through the body, some is scattered, and some is absorbed by cells within the body depending on the type and energy of the radiation. For purposes of this discussion, x-rays from fluoroscopic equipment and $\gamma$-rays from radionuclides are partially absorbed by the body, whereas energy from particulate radiation such as $\beta$ particles from radionuclides is totally absorbed by the body. Nearly all exposure in the perioperative environment is from x-rays, and a small amount of exposure is from $\gamma$-rays produced by radionuclides, mostly from patients who have had a nuclear medicine procedure. Physicists describe radiation dose in a variety of ways depending on the situation, but for purposes of occupational exposure, whole-body radiation dose is most commonly described and measured in terms of effective dose and measured in units of rem in the United States and sieverts (Sv) in the rest of the world. The effective dose is the average radiation dose to all body tissues exposed to the radiation weighted by the risk of stochastic effects to each tissue exposed to radiation.[6] When a single tissue is exposed (eg, skin), the radiation dose is not weighted for stochastic effects but is evaluated against regulatory dose limits for that tissue to protect against stochastic and deterministic effects.

## OBJECTIVES OF RADIATION PROTECTION

The specific objectives of radiation protection are to prevent the occurrence of clinically significant radiation-induced deterministic effects and to limit the likelihood of stochastic effects.[6] These objectives can be achieved by adhering to occupational dose limits established by regulatory agencies (**Table 1**) and by ensuring that occupational radiation exposures are as low as reasonably achievable (ALARA). These objectives are accomplished by implementation of a radiation safety program that uses facility design, shielding, procedures, training, and surveillance to keep radiation exposures ALARA.

**Table 1**
**Clinically significant deterministic effects can be prevented and stochastic effects limited by adhering to dose limits and practicing ALARA**

| Effect | Dose Threshold (rem) | Annual Dose Limit (rem) |
|---|---|---|
| Skin erythema (acute) | 300–600 | 50 |
| Cataracts | | |
|   Acute | 200 | 15 |
|   Chronic | 1000 | |
| In utero fetal effects | 10–20 | 0.5[a] |
| Cancer and leukemia | None established | 5 |

[a] Total during the pregnancy.

*Data from* National Council on Radiation Protection and Measurements. Limitation on exposure to ionizing radiation. NCRP report no. 116. Bethesda (MD): National Council on Radiation Protection and Measurements; 1993.

The person responsible for design of the radiation safety program is the radiation safety officer (RSO), who should be an individual with extensive training and education in areas such as radiation protection, radiation physics, radiation biology, instrumentation, dosimetry, and shielding design.[8] The RSO works with facilities personnel to design appropriate shielding in the walls of rooms where radiation is used to protect workers, patients, and the public. The RSO works with supervisors to develop procedures to ensure that workers are protected from radiation. The supervisor of a perioperative environment should contact the RSO for assistance whenever needed to refine practices and procedures and to assist in providing radiation safety training. Workers who have the potential to receive 25% of annual dose limits should be provided with appropriate dosimeters that measure radiation exposure.[8] Some states require personnel monitoring if workers could receive 10% of the limits. The RSO should be contacted to determine which workers need dosimeters and to provide the dosimeters.

## RADIATION EXPOSURE AND PROTECTION IN THE OPERATING ROOM

Use of less invasive surgical procedures and of new therapeutic methods has resulted in significant increases in the use of fluoroscopy in the operating room in the last few decades. For example, coronary angiography has become a common procedure, and its use along with angioplasty and coronary stent placement is often viewed as a lifesaving procedure that poses significantly less risk to the patient than open heart surgery. Although the use of radiological procedures has increased in recent years, the risks to medical personnel are minimal as long as radiation exposures are kept ALARA.

The greatest likelihood of occupational radiation exposure in the operating room occurs during fluoroscopy, particularly during interventional procedures. The dose received by medical workers depends on the type of procedure, the amount of fluoroscopic time, patient size, and other factors affected by the complexity of the operation. The actual source of radiation exposure to workers is not the fluoroscopy machine but the patient. Radiograph photons directed at the patient either pass through the patient and interact with the image receptor or they interact with the patient and table by 1 of 2 modes: photoelectric effect, in which the photon is totally absorbed, or Compton scattering, in which a portion of the photon energy is scattered in another direction. The scattered radiograph photons are the source of radiation exposure to workers. Therefore, workers are exposed to more radiation during procedures in which patients receive large doses of radiation. **Box 1** lists some of the procedures that often require extended fluoroscopic exposure time. Operating room personnel should pay particular attention to application of radiation safety principles during these procedures.

Workers in the operating room can limit their radiation exposure by application of 3 radiation safety principles: limiting time of exposure, increasing distance from the source, and using shielding. Because the fluoroscopic on-time is controlled by the operator (eg, radiologist or cardiologist), others in the room can control their exposure time only by avoiding exposure altogether (ie, avoid being in the room unless necessary). If their presence in the room is required, they should maximize their distance from the patient, wear protective lead (aprons and in some cases thyroid shields), and use protective lead barriers such as free-standing, clear, lead equivalent shields.

The intensity of the scattered radiation decreases with the square of the distance from the patient; therefore, radiation exposure drops dramatically by stepping back from the patient whenever possible. Radiation exposure 30 cm (1 ft) from the edge of the radiation field (side of the patient) is approximately 1% of the exposure at the entrance of the patient. Increasing the distance to 1 m decreases the exposure to 0.1% (1 m = 3.3 ft, $3.3^2$ = 10, 1% ÷ 10 = 0.1%). Therefore, if a patient received an entrance exposure of 1 rem, a nurse standing at the side of the patient during the procedure would have received 0.01 rem at 30 cm (1 ft) or 0.001 rem at 1 m from the patient.

Most states require anyone who is in a fluoroscopic room during exposure to wear a 0.5-mm lead equivalent apron. Depending on the energy of the fluoroscopic x-rays, a 0.5-mm lead apron will attenuate 95% to 98% of the scattered radiation. Lead aprons are particularly effective at reducing exposure from x-rays but not from radionuclides, which typically emit more energetic radiation (**Fig. 1**). If a patient receives a skin dose of 1 rem during fluoroscopy, a worker who is wearing a lead apron (assume 95% attenuation) and standing 1 m from the side of the patient would receive a dose under the apron of 0.5% of the entrance dose or 0.0005 × 1 rem = 0.0005 rem. For purposes of comparison, people in the United States receive a dose of approximately 0.3 rem per year from background radiation including radon and approximately 0.002 rem from cosmic radiation during a 4-hour airplane flight.[9]

---

**Box 1**
**Some procedures that often require extended fluoroscopic exposure times**

Biliary or abscess drainage or stone removal

Embolization procedures

Endoscopic retrograde cholangiography

Genitourinary procedures

Percutaneous transluminal angioplasty

Percutaneous transhepatic cholangiography

Percutaneous nephrostomy

Radiofrequency catheter ablation

Stent placement

Thrombolytic and fibrinolytic procedures

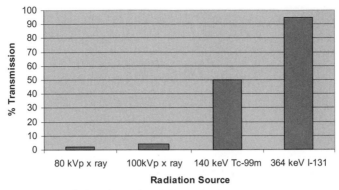

**Fig. 1.** Percentage transmission through a 0.5-mm lead apron.

## RADIATION EXPOSURE AND PROTECTION OUTSIDE THE OPERATING ROOM

Patients exposed to x-rays are not made radioactive, so health care personnel who work with these patients are not exposed to radiation except during fluoroscopy in the operating room or fluoroscopy suite. On the other hand, patients who receive nuclear medicine imaging studies are radioactive because they are injected with radio-pharmaceuticals. Examples of typical radiation exposure rates from nuclear medicine patients are shown in **Table 2**. Except for heart scans and positron emission tomography (PET) scans the exposures are low. The exposure rates from heart scans and PET scans are similar to those from hyperthyroid patients treated with radioiodine. However, the radioactive and biologic half-lives for radioiodine are longer than for the radionuclides used in diagnostic scans. Therefore, nurses who care for radioiodine patients are trained by the RSO or designee on how to minimize time and maximize distance when caring for radioiodine patients. For example, distance can be maximized by talking to the patient from the doorway rather than the bedside to determine how well the patient is feeling.

| Table 2 Typical radiation exposure rates from nuclear medicine patients | |
| --- | --- |
| **Nuclear Medicine Study** | **Millirem/h at 1 m[a]** |
| Diagnostic scans | |
| Indium scan (4 mCi [111]In) | 0.3 |
| Gallium scan (3 mCi [67]Ga) | 0.35 |
| Bone scan (20 mCi [99m]Tc) | 0.9 |
| Sestimibi heart scan (30 mCi [99m]Tc) | 14 |
| Thallium heart scan (4 mCi [201]Tl) | 3 |
| PET scan (10 mCi [18]F) | 2.9 |
| Therapeutic applications | |
| Hyperthyroid treatment (10 mCi [131]I) | 1.5–2 |
| Thyroid cancer treatment (100 mCi [131]I) | 15–20 |

[a] Radiation exposure 1 m from patient shortly after injection of the radiopharmaceutical (1 millirem = 0.001 rem).

Most patients are not subject to invasive procedures immediately following a nuclear medicine examination. Surgeries usually need to be scheduled and take place after the radiopharmaceutical has either undergone complete radioactive decay, or elimination from the body, or both. An exception to the usual is sentinel lymphadenectomy for breast cancer or melanoma, which may take place later the same day as the imaging of the sentinel lymph node. The radiation dose to the surgeon's hand during sentinel lymphadenectomy is approximately 0.01 rem for breast cancer and 0.002 rem for melanoma.[10] These doses are low compared with the regulatory dose limits (see **Table 1**). Radiation dose to pathology staff who handle these specimens is lower than to the surgeon because of the short time spent handling the specimens. The Surgical Pathology Committee of the College of American Pathologists has developed recommendations for specimen handling, labeling, transportation, and processing, which should be followed to prevent radioactive contamination and to keep radiation exposures ALARA.[9]

Brachytherapy is the use of sealed sources of radionuclides to treat cancer. Brachytherapy involves temporary or permanent implantation of sealed sources in or near the tumor. Perhaps the most common use of sealed sources to treat patients in the perioperative environment is permanent implantation of iodine 125 ($^{125}I$) in the form of small sealed sources in the shape of small rods often called seeds (**Fig. 2**), and the most common treatment with $^{125}I$ seeds is brachytherapy for prostate cancer. For prostate implants, patients are anesthetized and prepared in an operating room or brachytherapy suite. A plastic template is placed near the perineum of the patient and an intrarectal ultrasound probe is placed in the rectum to image the prostate during implantation of the $^{125}I$ seeds. The template is used to position needles that contain the seeds. Wearing a lead apron, the radiation oncologist or urologist injects the seeds into the prostate in a prescribed fashion to deliver a high dose of radiation to the prostate gland. Often fluoroscopy is used in conjunction with the ultrasound to image the prostate during brachytherapy treatment and is the main source of radiation exposure to operating staff participating in these implants.[11] The radiograph

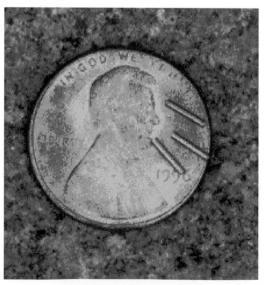

**Fig. 2.** $^{125}I$ brachytherapy seeds used to treat prostate cancer.

technologist, surgical technician, and nurse, if required to be in the room, wear a lead apron and stand at least a meter (several feet) from the patient to minimize their radiation exposure. The radiation dose received by the physician's dosimeter worn at the collar outside the lead apron ranges from approximately 0.007 to 0.015 rem per patient.[11] After the seeds are implanted the patient is placed in a recovery room for several hours and then dismissed. In some cases the patient is hospitalized overnight. Because the energy of the $^{125}$I photons is low, on the order of 30 keV compared with 365 keV for photons from $^{131}$I, the radiation exposure rate is only approximately 0.001 rem/h at 1 m from the patient.

Another common application of temporary implants is $^{125}$I eye plaques for the treatment of ocular melanoma. A physicist fixes several $^{125}$I seeds into an eye plaque, which an eye surgeon then sutures over the lesion. The plaque is left in place for several days to irradiate the cancer cells. The eye plaque contains a backing made of gold or silver to reduce the radiation exposure to other tissues of the patient. This backing and an eye patch reduce the radiation exposure rate at 1 m from the patient to nearly background. Thus, health care personnel receive no measurable radiation exposure from patients with eye plaques.

Some temporary brachytherapy implants use the radionuclide $^{192}$Ir, which emits several different γ-rays with energies in the range of 296 to 604 keV. Because these γ-ray photons are energetic, patients must be hospitalized in specifically designated hospital rooms to protect health care staff, other patients, and members of the public. These patients are taken to surgery to have catheters placed in or near the tumor. Then the patients are moved to their hospital room where the radiation oncologist inserts plastic tubes into the catheters, which contain $^{192}$Ir spaced in a prescribed fashion to deliver an optimal radiation dose to the tumor. Nurses who care for these patients receive specific instruction from the RSO, radiation oncologist, or physicist on how to minimize their time with the patient, how to maximize distance, and how to use a bedside shield to keep their radiation exposure to a low level. Nurses are also trained in how to recognize when the $^{192}$Ir ribbon has been dislodged by the patient and are instructed to call the radiation oncologist immediately if the placement of the ribbon seems to have been changed.

Some procedures involve the administration of liquid radioactivity to a cavity in the body (eg, a brain cyst to irradiate a tumor boundary or the abdominal cavity to irradiate ovarian tumor cells). The radionuclides most commonly used for these purposes are $^{32}$P and $^{125}$I. $^{32}$P emits a β particle; therefore, all the radiation energy is absorbed within the body of the patient. Most of the radiation dose from the low-energy $^{125}$I photons is absorbed within the body of the patient. Consequently, there is little concern for external radiation exposure to health care personnel from these patients. However, it is possible for the liquid radioactive solution to leak from the administration site. Nurses must be instructed to watch for this leakage and, if leakage is observed, to place pressure on the site of administration to stop leakage and to report the leakage to the appropriate radiation physician and RSO. It is important that action be taken quickly to prevent radioactive contamination from being tracked out of the patient's hospital room. Internal contamination of nurses can be prevented by practicing standard precautions while caring for these patients, including hand washing immediately after leaving the patient room.

## ASSOCIATION OF OPERATING ROOM NURSES RECOMMENDED PRACTICES

The Association of Operating Room Nurses (AORN) has developed a set of recommended radiation safety practices as guidelines adaptable to various practice settings.[12] These settings include operating rooms, ambulatory surgery centers, physicians' offices, cardiac catheterization rooms, endoscopy suites, radiology and interventional radiology departments, and other areas where operative and other invasive procedures may be performed. A summary and discussion of the AORN recommended practices as they apply to occupational radiation exposure is provided here. The reader is referred to the AORN recommended practices for a full understanding of the recommendations.

I. The patient's exposure to radiation should be minimized: as discussed earlier, keeping the patient radiation dose as low as possible also reduces the radiation exposure to medical staff.

II. The patient should be protected from unnecessary radiation exposure: in addition to optimizing patient care (eg, keeping extraneous patient body parts out of the radiation beam to prevent injury), reducing the amount of body tissue in the beam also reduces radiation scatter. Anything that can be done to reduce scatter reduces occupational exposure.

III. Occupational exposure to radiation should be minimized: this recommendation is accomplished by application of the principles of time, distance, and shielding as discussed earlier. Although the needs of the patient should come first, vigilant application of these principles during the care of patients keeps occupational exposure ALARA.

IV. Shielding devices should be handled carefully, visually examined before use, and radiographed at least annually to detect and prevent damage that could diminish their effectiveness: health care institutions implement this recommendation in a variety of ways, wherein the department that owns the lead aprons, the radiology department, the RSO, a consultant or vendor, or some other responsible party performs a fluoroscopy examination on the lead aprons annually and records that the examination was completed. If the examination indicates that the integrity of the apron is intact, the apron is approved for continued use. If a hole in the apron is discovered, the apron is taken out of use and discarded in an approved lead recycling program.

V. Individuals should be protected from exposure to patients who have received diagnostic or therapeutic radionuclides that may pose a radiation risk: as shown in **Table 2**, the exposure rate from patients who have received diagnostic radionuclides is low. The exposure rate to health care workers and the public as these patients travel through the clinic or hospital is low enough that no special precautions are necessary. These patients can be roomed anywhere in the hospital without special precautions. However, care of patients who have been treated with [131]I or temporary brachytherapy implants requires special precautions to prevent unnecessary radiation exposure to health care personnel and to other patients. These patients must be hospitalized in rooms specifically identified for that purpose, and health care personnel must receive specific instructions on how to minimize their own occupational exposure while caring for these patients. Instructions should address how to minimize time, maximize distance, and use portable bedside shields while caring for these patients. Contamination control measures are important in radioiodine rooms and should include disposable floor covering to facilitate decontamination of the room after the patient is dismissed. Caregivers should practice standard precautions when caring for these patients to reduce the risk of internal contamination.

VI. Radiation monitors or dosimeters should be worn by personnel who are in frequent proximity to radiation as determined by the radiation safety officer: as indicated in the earlier discussion, regulations require that any worker whose occupational radiation exposure may exceed 10% of the occupational dose limit (see **Table 1**) must be provided with personnel monitoring such as a dosimeter. During fluoroscopy the dosimeter should be worn at the collar level outside the lead apron. When a dosimeter is provided to monitor the abdominal dose during pregnancy, it should be worn at the waist under the lead apron. A ring badge that is provided to monitor hand dose during operations such as administration of radiopharmaceuticals should be worn in a manner that registers the highest radiation dose to the hand. Badges should be exchanged and cared for in accordance with instructions provided by the RSO.

VII. Therapeutic radiation sources should be handled minimally to minimize exposure. Protective measures are implemented to prevent injury: therapeutic radiation sources normally are handled only by or under the supervision of radiation oncology and nuclear medicine personnel who have been trained to handle them safely. However, nurses who care for patients who have been treated with therapeutic radionuclides must be trained in emergency response to deal with issues such as a radioiodine patient who vomits shortly after receiving [131]I or a disoriented brachytherapy patient who dislodges a brachytherapy implant. The RSO, radiation oncologist, nuclear medicine physician, or designee should provide this training.[13]

VIII. Measures taken to protect patients during the procedure from the risks of direct and indirect radiation exposure should be documented on the perioperative nursing record: this documentation is beneficial in promoting continuity of care and facilitating communication during hand-off of patients between shifts. The documentation should also include any special instructions such as monitoring the position of a brachytherapy catheter.

IX. Policies and procedures regarding radiation exposure should be written, reviewed periodically, and readily available within the practice setting: there are many operations within the perioperative environment in which teamwork provides synergy in assuring a safe environment of care. Development of radiation policies and procedures for a particular practice is an activity in which all disciplines should recognize each other's expertise and work together to develop the best procedures for the benefit of the patient and the caregiver. Perioperative personnel, the RSO, and radiation medicine staff need to work together to maximize patient benefit and minimize radiation exposure to health care personnel.

X. Personnel should receive initial education, training, and competency validation and at least annual updates on new regulations and procedures: in some cases personnel receive this training during their formal education (eg, radiography school). In other cases, additional specific radiation safety training is necessary (eg, nurses who care for patients hospitalized with temporary brachytherapy implants). In the second case training should include some hands-on training to provide health care personnel with some operational experience before on-the-job training that includes care of a radiation patient. In both cases annual updates are important to provide all personnel with changes in standards and regulations as well as any new information on how to keep their radiation exposures ALARA.

XI. Only personnel who have received specific state-approved radiological training may be permitted to operate radiographic equipment. States now require licensure of personnel who operate radiographic equipment. For this reason and for the safety of patients and health care personnel, only licensed personnel, physicists, and authorized repair personnel should operate radiographic machines. Only licensed practitioners of the healing arts (eg, physicians and nurse practitioners) should operate fluoroscopic equipment unless the hospital or radiographic facility has received specific approval from the state radiation control agency to allow licensed radiographers to operate fluoroscopic equipment under the direction of a licensed practitioner.

## SUMMARY

Radiation is an important tool in the diagnosis and treatment of numerous medical conditions. Personnel in the perioperative environment must be trained in how to recognize operations during which they could be exposed to radiation and how to minimize their exposure. The operations most likely to result in potentially high radiation exposures are fluoroscopy in operating and procedure rooms and therapeutic applications of radionuclides. Other procedures that use radiation including nuclear medicine result in low or no measurable radiation doses to perioperative personnel. However, personnel who are exposed to measurable radiation doses, even if they are below the levels that require personal dosimetry monitoring, should receive periodic (eg, annual) updates on radiation procedures, standards, and regulations to help them to keep their radiation exposures ALARA.

## REFERENCES

1. Bursik SM, Vetter RJ. Professor Roentgen's discovery of x rays. Health Phys 1991; 60:132.
2. United Nations Scientific Committee on the Effects of Atomic Radiation. UNSCEAR 2006 Report: effects of ionizing radiation. Volume 1: Report to the General Assembly, Scientific Annexes A and B. New York: United Nations; 2008.
3. Committee to Assess Health Risks from Exposure to Low Levels of Ionizing Radiation. Health risks from exposure to low levels of ionizing radiation. BEIR VII Phase 2. Washington, DC: The National Academies Press; 2006.
4. March HC. Leukemia in radiologists. Radiology 1944;43:275–8.
5. Yoshinaga S, Mabuchi K, Sigurdson A, et al. Cancer risk among radiologists and radiologic technologists; review of epidemiologic studies. Radiology 2004;233: 313–21.
6. National Council on Radiation Protection and Measurements. Limitation on exposure to ionizing radiation. NCRP report no. 116. Bethesda (MD): National Council on Radiation Protection and Measurements; 1993.
7. Ainsbury EA, Bouffler SD, Dorr W, et al. Radiation cataractogenesis: a review of recent studies. Radiat Res 2009;172:1–9.
8. National Council on Radiation Protection and Measurements. Radiation protection for medical and allied health personnel. NCRP report no. 105. Bethesda (MD): National Council on Radiation Protection and Measurements; 1989.
9. National Council on Radiation Protection and Measurements. Ionizing radiation exposure of the population of the United States. NCRP report no. 160. Bethesda (MD): National Council on Radiation Protection and Measurements; 2009.
10. Fitzgibbons PL, Livolsi VA, Surgical Pathology Committee of the College of American Pathologists. Recommendations for handling radioactive specimens obtained by sentinel lymphadenectomy. Am J Surg Pathol 2000;24(11):1549–51.
11. Schwartz DJ, Davis BJ, Vetter RJ, et al. Radiation exposure to operating room personnel during transperineal interstitial permanent prostate brachytherapy. Brachytherapy 2003;2:98–102.

12. Association of Operating Room Nurses. Recommended practices for reducing radiological exposure in the perioperative practice setting. AORN J 2007;85(5): 989–1002.

13. National Council on Radiation Protection and Measurements. Management of radionuclide therapy patients. NCRP report no. 155. Bethesda (MD): National Council on Radiation Protection and Measurements; 2006.

# Overview of Embolotherapy: Agents, Indications, Applications, and Nursing Management

Sandra L. Schwaner, MSN, ACNP-BC[a,b,*], Stephen B. Haug, RTR, CV[c], Alan H. Matsumoto, MD, FSIR[d]

**KEYWORDS**

- Embolotherapy • Embolization • Tumor • Bleeding
- Nursing management • Complications

Early interventional radiology was often called angiography or special procedures and was seen as a purely diagnostic tool for mapping lymphatics, veins and arteries, bile ducts, and urinary system for surgeons. As balloons, stents, and embolic agents were devised, this specialty has moved from being diagnostic to being treatment oriented using image-guided catheter-directed techniques. Much of interventional radiology focuses on 1 of the 2 outcomes: vascular embolization or the cessation of blood flow to a target area, and percutaneous transluminal angioplasty and stenting or the restoring of blood, bile, or urine flow to or from an end organ.[1] This article focuses on the many uses of vascular embolization in medicine today as well as the specific embolic agents currently available, how and why they are used, and types of procedures in which each would be valuable. The role of the nurse in evaluating and caring for the patient before, during, and after an embolization procedure is discussed. An explanation of some of the common complications, how to recognize and treat them, and a brief discussion of the future of embolization and interventional radiology is also provided.

[a] APN1 Department of Interventional Radiology, Division of Radiology, University of Virginia Health System, PO Box 800377, Charlottesville, VA, USA
[b] Department of Radiology, Division of Interventional Radiology, PO Box 800377, Charlottesville, VA 22908-0377, USA
[c] Tegtmeyer School of Angio/Interventional Radiology, Division of Radiology, University of Virginia Health System, PO Box 800377, Charlottesville, VA 22908-0377, USA
[d] Division of Radiology, UVA CORS, University of Virginia Health System, PO Box 800170, Charlottesville, VA 22908-0170, USA
* Corresponding author. Department of Radiology, Division of Interventional Radiology, PO Box 800377, Charlottesville, VA 22908-0377.
E-mail address: sls5c@virginia.edu

Perioperative Nursing Clinics 5 (2010) 137–176
doi:10.1016/j.cpen.2010.02.006
1556-7931/10/$ – see front matter © 2010 Elsevier Inc. All rights reserved.

An embolic event blocks blood flow in a vessel or vessels, reducing perfusion to an end organ. Embolization as a procedure is the deliberate creation of an embolic event.[1] Embolization must be carefully controlled to achieve the desired effects while reducing complications. Vessels can be embolized to control excessive or unwanted bleeding,[2–9] to reduce symptoms caused by a tumor[10–14] or vascular malformation,[15–19] to devascularize a tumor in preparation for surgical removal,[20–25] or for treatment of inoperable vascular tumors.[26–31] Determining the type and specific embolic agent to be used depends on several criteria that are discussed later in this article.

## EMBOLIC AGENTS

Embolic agents can be divided into 2 categories: temporary agents and permanent agents (**Table 1**). Temporary agents obstruct blood flow but then dissolve or are eliminated by the immune system within a defined period of time, usually about 2 to 6 weeks.[1] Temporary embolic agents are used to allow healing of injured vessels or to provide a window for patient stabilization before more definitive surgical repair, without permanent obstruction of blood flow to the end organ. Permanent agents are designed to provide irreversible obstruction of blood flow to the targeted lesion or end organ.[32] Every embolic agent has its advantages and limitations. Various embolic agents and their indications for use, contraindications, and deployment considerations are described here.

### Temporary Embolic Agents

#### Autologous agents

In the 1970s, because of the lack of availability of premanufactured agents, autologous materials were the first embolic agents used to occlude bleeding vessels.[33,34] Clotted blood, fat, muscle, and connective tissue were the most common autologous agents used.[35] These materials could easily be obtained from the patient, with minimal cost; however, they required harvesting and preparation before embolization. The most common agent used was autologous blood clot,[34] but it had a high incidence of fibrinolytic breakdown and vessel recanalization with reperfusion within hours of the procedure.[35] Absorbable gelatin sponge has replaced autologous clot as the embolic agent of choice,[1] although autologous agents are still being used in developing countries where financial constraints limit the availability of synthetic embolic agents.

#### Resorbable gelatin sponge agents

Absorbable gelatin sponge Gelfoam (Pfizer, Inc, New York, NY, USA) or Surgifoam (Johnson & Johnson, Inc, Warrenton, NJ, USA) was introduced as a topical agent in 1945 to aid in obtaining hemostasis during surgical procedures.[35] It is biodegradable but remains intact in vivo for several weeks to months.

Gelfoam is packaged in 2 forms: powder and sheet or block.[1,36] The powder particles are approximately 40 to 60 μm in size.[36] This allows for embolization of small arterial branches but increases the risk of tissue ischemia or necrosis. Precision in administration of Gelfoam powder to the target of choice is essential.[36] The block or sheet of Gelfoam can be cut into particles, pledgets, or torpedoes, or made into a slurry to customize its size for the target vessels.[1,34] Gelfoam is used to stop hemorrhage from injured vessels, allowing the vessels to heal and eventually recanalize over time.[37]

The primary complications associated with the use of Gelfoam are related to nontarget embolization (occluding an artery that should have been left open), tissue infarction due to use of particles too small in size (seen most often with use of Gelfoam

**Table 1**
Categories of embolic agents

| Type of Embolic Agent | Embolic Material | Indication | Points to Remember |
|---|---|---|---|
| Temporary agents | Autologous agents | Stop blood flow | Inexpensive, but high risk of breakdown and recanalization |
| | Resorbable gelatin sponge | Temporary control of small or large vessels | Can be administered as powder or slurry. Beware distal embolization with ischemia. Recanalization in 4–6 weeks |
| Permanent agents | | | |
| Solid agents | Coils | Aneurysms, large vessel occlusion, complete occlusion | Many sizes and shapes available, must pair appropriate coil with defect |
| | Plugs | Complete occlusion of larger vessel with minimal product | Careful sizing essential, follow manufacturer instructions closely. Use often mixed with coils and particles to achieve thrombosis |
| | Detachable balloons | Permanent large vessel occlusion | Rarely used in United States, because of availability of coils and plugs |
| Particulate agents | PVA (polyvinyl alcohol) | Single or multiple small vessel occlusion | Many sizes available. Careful administration essential to avoid catheter occlusion or nontarget embolization |
| | Compressible microspheres | Often used in UAE, TACE, for occlusion of multiple small vessels | Sizing is important, some brands cause less inflammation, more expensive than standard PVA embolization |
| Liquid agents | Thrombin | Treatment of pseudoaneurysms, soak coils before deployment | Inject carefully to prevent reflux and inadvertent distal embolization |
| | Dehydrated alcohol | Devascularization of renal cell carcinoma before surgery, treatment of vascular malformations | Prevention of reflux and leakage essential. Can be painful. Many patients require anesthesia |
| | Sodium tetradecyl sulfate | Occlusion of surface varicosities, vascular malformations | More forgiving to surrounding tissue than alcohol, can be injected as foam |
| | Glues | Treatment of AVMs, endoleaks, gastric varices | Care must be taken so that catheter does not become imbedded in the glue. Inject carefully and rapidly |
| | Onyx | Treatment of AVMs, endoleaks, gastric varices | Proven safe in contact with graft material. Inject slowly |

*Abbreviations*: AVM, arterial-venous malformation; TACE, transarterial chemoembolization; UAE, uterine artery embolization.

powder), incomplete control of bleeding due to inadequate embolization, or incomplete tissue healing (ie, an ulcer) before degradation of the Gelfoam in vivo.[5,32,34]

## Permanent Embolic Agents

Permanent agents are designed to remain in place for the whole life of the patient (see **Table 1**). Permanent agents can be divided into 3 broad categories: nonliquid nonparticulate, particulate, and liquid embolic agents.

### Nonparticulate, nonliquid agents

Nonparticulate agents include coils, plugs, and detachable balloons. One of the most commonly used permanent embolic agents is the metal coil. The first coil was designed by Gianturco and Wallace in 1975. It was constructed of a steel coil guidewire with the inner mandril (core) removed and wool fibers entwined in the steel coil.[32,38] These fibers increased the thrombogenicity of the coil.[35] Eventually, the wool fiber was supplanted by a polyester (Dacron) fiber material because the wool fibers produced a severe granulomatous arteritis in the adventitia of the artery.[35] Coils are currently available in materials ranging from platinum and stainless steel to a new material inconel, a nickel-chromium-based alloy (**Fig. 1**).

Coils come in a variety of sizes, shapes, lengths, materials, and deployment mechanisms (detachable or pushable).[32,34] Coils are further subdivided according to whether they are coated with any added material (ie, fibers or hydrogels) to increase their thrombogenicity. Detachable coils (**Figs. 2** and **3**) are attached to a guidewire and then released in a controlled fashion once the position of the coil is felt to be satisfactory. If positioning of the coil is not optimal, the coil can be recaptured and repositioned before its release. Retrieving a coil once it has been deployed is difficult. Pushable coils are pushed through the catheter to the target vessel, but once they exit the catheter they are released and cannot be repositioned.

The most conformable coil material constructed today is platinum. Historically, platinum was obtained by cutting coronary guidewires and injecting the small platinum wire fragments through a microcatheter to the target vessel.[35] This early discovery determined that platinum was extremely biocompatible, very radiopaque, and somewhat thrombogenic. In addition, platinum is a nonferrous material, so it is magnetic resonance (MR) imaging compatible.[32] Fibrous materials such as silk and Dacron were added to the platinum coil to increase its thrombogenicity.[32] Many different companies produce an assortment of coil shapes and configurations, from the basic

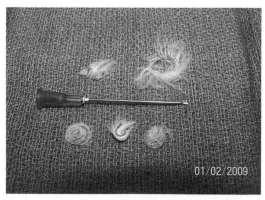

**Fig. 1.** Multiple sized coils shown in comparison to a standard 19-gauge 1.5-in needle.

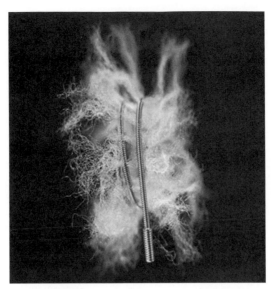

**Fig. 2.** The MReye coil (Cook Medical, Inc, Bloomington, IN, USA). This coil, constructed of inconel material, part of the family of nickel-chromium-based alloys, increases visibility and radial strength. It is also magnetic resonance (MR) compatible and is available in pushable and detachable forms.

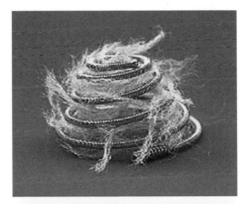

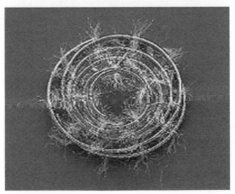

**Fig. 3.** Tornado coils (Cook Medical, Inc, Bloomington, IN, USA).

helical shape (**Figs. 3** and **4**) to complex shapes (**Fig. 5**). In addition, these fibered coils come in different wire diameters; 0.018-in coils for use with microcatheters and 0.035-in coils for use with larger diagnostic catheters.[32]

Platinum coils are available in pushable and detachable versions. Traditionally, detachable coils were primarily used to treat intracranial aneurysms. The first-generation detachable coil was nonfibered, noncoated, and helical shaped, and called the Guglielmi detachable coil (GDC) (see **Figs. 4** and **5**). Today, some detachable coils have fibers (Interlock; Boston Scientific, Natick, MA, USA). The Interlock is a 0.018-in platinum microcoil system that can be used with microcatheters for the embolization of different pathologies, including aneurysms and arteriovenous fistulas (**Fig. 6**). The Flipper coil (Cook Medical, Inc, Bloomington, IN, USA) is a 0.035-in detachable platinum coil system. It has a threaded locking mechanism, so that once the coil is

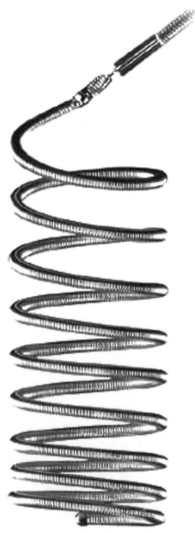

**Fig. 4.** Guglielmi detachable coil (GDC 2).

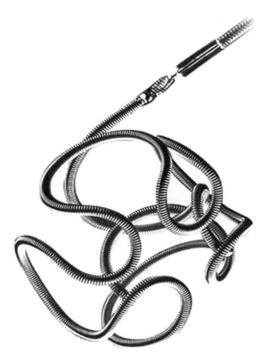

**Fig. 5.** GDC 360° coil. Today, the GDC coil is manufactured in many different styles, from complex shape GDC 360° to GDC 3-dimensional shape, yet their primary purpose of aneurysm coiling has not changed.

placed within the vessel, the delivery cable wire is rotated, releasing the coil from the cable (**Fig. 7**).

The HydroCoil (MicroVention, Inc, Minneapolis, MN, USA) is a detachable platinum coil. It contains a dehydrated polymer (**Fig. 8**) that begins to expand on contact with an ionic solution (blood or saline) (**Fig. 9**). The advantage of this type of coil is twofold.

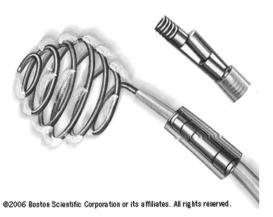

**Fig. 6.** Tornado Coil manufactured by Boston Scientific. (*Courtesy of* Boston Scientific, Inc, Natick, MA, USA; with permission.)

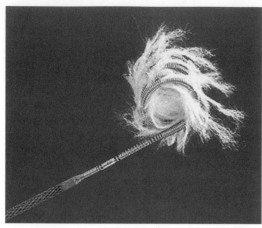

**Fig. 7.** Flipper coil (Cook Medical, Inc, Bloomington, IN, USA). Advanced via a 0.35-in guidewire.

First, the HydroCoil consumes space. It expands to 6 times its size over time within the target vessel so that fewer coils are required to create a vascular occlusion. The second advantage is that the HydroCoil provides a matrix on which fibroblastic cells can grow leading to permanent occlusion of the aneurysm. Thus, the vessel grows endothelial cells across the hydrocoil, mimicking the internal wall of the vessel and eliminating further chance of aneurysm filling.

Recently, detachable vascular plugs have become available as an alternative to coils. The AMPLATZER Vascular Plug (AVP I and II; AGA Medical Corporation, Minneapolis, MN, USA) is made of a very fine nitinol wire mesh that obstructs the blood flow through the intended vessel and induces thrombosis of the target vessel.[1,32]

Case study 1. The AMPLATZER Vascular Plug was used to provide large vessel occlusion. A patient with descending thoracic aortic aneurysm needed distal thoracic stent graft, requiring coverage of vessels off the aorta. There was concern about refilling and endoleak development. For this reason the decision was made to preemptively embolize celiac artery (patient with patent superior mesenteric artery and inferior mesenteric artery) (**Figs. 10–12**).

Nitinol is a thermal-memory alloy of nickel and titanium. Once exposed to body temperature, the AVP tries to take its predetermined shape. The plug is mounted on a threaded positioning cable and is preloaded into a sheath. The AVP is pushed from its sheath into the prepositioned guide catheter or sheath using its positioning

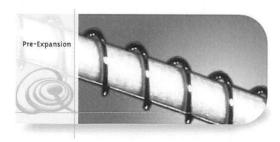

Pre-Expansion

**Fig. 8.** Hydrocoil preexpansion.

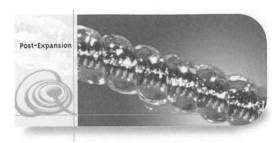

**Fig. 9.** Hydrocoil (the same as in **Fig. 8**) postexpansion, after contact with blood.

cable and then pushed through the guiding sheath/catheter into the target vessel. Once in its desired position, the guide catheter/sheath is retracted and the AVP is exposed and expands within the target vessel. If the AVP is in a satisfactory location, the positioning cable is rotated to unscrew it from the AVP, thus releasing the AVP. If the AVP is in an undesirable location, then the delivery catheter/sheath can be advanced to recapture and, if necessary, to remove the AVP. Currently, the AVP can be purchased in 2 forms: the first-generation AVP I device (**Fig. 13**) and the second-generation AVP II device (**Fig. 14**). The AVP II has a finer mesh and greater surface area, and has been shown to cause more rapid vascular occlusion when compared with the AVP I device. However, the AVP II is longer than the AVP I device and needs a longer vascular segment in which to be deployed.

Delivering the AVP requires careful sizing (**Fig. 15**). The plug size is determined by the diameter of the intended vessel, but the size of the plug should be larger than the diameter of the vessel to allow the sides of the plug to be flushed up against the vessel wall. Each plug is designed to fit through a particular size-guiding sheath or catheter. The first-generation plug should be 30% to 50% larger than the vessel, whereas the second generation only requires 20% to 30% oversizing. The plug

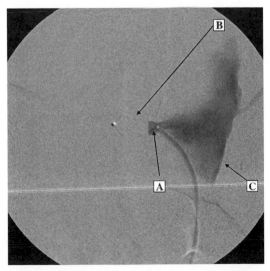

**Fig. 10.** Lateral projection of AMPLATZER I in the celiac axis. (A) Injection of the occluded celiac artery. (B) AMPLATZER itself before deployment. (C) Diseased thoracic aorta.

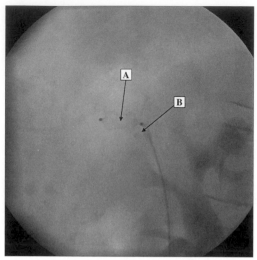

**Fig. 11.** Magnified image of AMPLATZER within the celiac vessel. (A) AMPLATZER Plug. (B) Connecting catheter.

diameter then determines the size of sheath/catheter needed for proper deployment of the plug. A third- and fourth-generation AVP is currently being developed.[1,34]

Although detachable balloons have been used in the past for embolization procedures, their use has markedly diminished. The use of detachable balloons has largely been supplanted by the use of the AVP and detachable HydroCoils.[32]

### Particulate agents

Particulate embolic agents have been used for many years to treat various vascular diseases and can be divided into 2 major categories: polyvinyl alcohol (PVA) and synthetic microspheres.

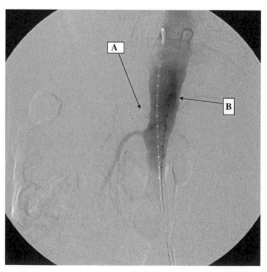

**Fig. 12.** Postprocedure injection. (A) Vascular plug and occlusion are present beyond the celiac axis. (B) Diseased aorta ready for treatment with endovascular stent graft.

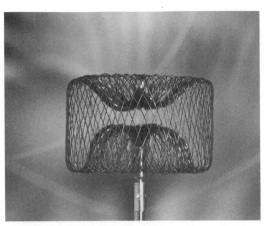

**Fig. 13.** AMPLATZER Vascular Plug. This was the original vascular plug.

PVA is manufactured and packaged in various sizes and shapes. In the 1970s, before its availability as a manufactured embolic agent, interventional radiologists (IRs) were making PVA particles themselves by placing styrofoam packaging material from furniture and stereo equipment into a blender, fragmenting the styrofoam (made from PVA), packaging the various-sized particles into a container, and then sterilizing it in an autoclave. The particles were then used empirically as a more permanent agent to embolize tumors. Control of the size of the particles was somewhat crude. In the 1980s, the industry began making medical-grade PVA particles and the technology has gradually been further refined (Alan H. Matsumoto, MD, Charlottesville VA, personal communication, 2009). The manufactured PVA particles are now prepackaged in a range of sizes, from 45 μm to larger than 1000 μm. Microscopically, traditional PVA particles resemble the shape of popcorn (**Fig. 16**), but PVA can now be manufactured in a spherical form as well (Boston Scientific, Natick, MA, USA; Angio-Dynamics, Queensbury, NY, USA) (**Fig. 17**).[1,2,6,7,10,13,18]

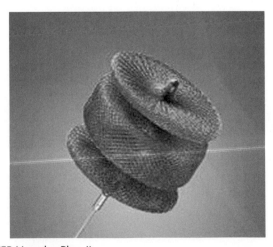

**Fig. 14.** AMPLATZER Vascular Plug II.

| AMPLATZER® Vascular Plug II<br>The Singular Solution for Rapid¹ Embolization Technology | | | | | | |
| --- | --- | --- | --- | --- | --- | --- |
| | | | **DELIVERY SYSTEM MINIMUM REQUIREMENTS** | | | |
| AMPLATZER<br>Vascular Plug II<br>Order Number | AMPLATZER<br>Vascular Plug II<br>Diameter (mm) | Pre-Implanted<br>Device<br>Length (mm) | **Sheath**<br>Minimum Size | Minimum ID<br>Required<br>(inches) | **Guide<br>Catheter**<br>Minimum Size | Maximum<br>Length<br>(cm) |
| 9-AVP2-003 | 3 | 6 | 4 Fr | 0.056" | 5 Fr | 100 |
| 9-AVP2-004 | 4 | 6 | 4 Fr | 0.056" | 5 Fr | 100 |
| 9-AVP2-006 | 6 | 6 | 4 Fr | 0.056" | 5 Fr | 100 |
| 9-AVP2-008 | 8 | 7 | 4 Fr | 0.056" | 5 Fr | 100 |
| 9-AVP2-010 | 10 | 7 | 5 Fr | 0.070" | 6 Fr | 100 |
| 9-AVP2-012 | 12 | 9 | 5 Fr | 0.070" | 6 Fr | 100 |
| 9-AVP2-014 | 14 | 10 | 6 Fr | 0.086" | 8 Fr | 100 |
| 9-AVP2-016 | 16 | 12 | 6 Fr | 0.086" | 8 Fr | 100 |
| 9-AVP2-018 | 18 | 14 | 7 Fr | 0.098" | 9 Fr | 100 |
| 9-AVP2-020 | 20 | 16 | 7 Fr | 0.098" | 9 Fr | 100 |
| 9-AVP2-022 | 22 | 18 | 7 Fr | 0.098" | 9 Fr | 100 |

**Fig. 15.** Sizing guide for AMPLATZER plugs. (*Courtesy of* AGA Medical Corporation, Plymouth, MN, USA; with permission.)

Once deployed into an artery, PVA provokes an inflammatory and dense fibrous connective tissue reaction.[36] The particle size is chosen based on the treatment goal and level of embolization desired. The most common size of PVA is 500 μm.[1,36] However, sizes as small as 150 μm are used in many malignant tumor embolization procedures because they provide a greater distal embolization, with less chance of revascularization and greater chance for tumor infarction.[26–30]

The process of administering PVA begins with mixing the PVA with either full-strength contrast, or a one-to-one mixture of normal saline and contrast in a glass

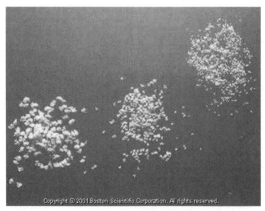

**Fig. 16.** Various sizes of PVA particles. (*Courtesy of* Boston Scientific, Inc, Natick, MA, USA; with permission.)

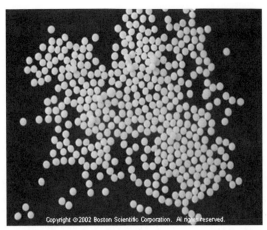

**Fig. 17.** Spherical PVA particles (often referred to as "microspheres"). (*Courtesy of* Boston Scientific, Inc, Natick, MA, USA; with permission.)

shot glass on a separate sterile embolization table. The use of the separate table reduces the chance for inadvertent mixing up of embolization syringes with contrast and flush syringes. In addition, labels are used to identify each size of PVA for all shot glasses and syringes.[36] PVA tends to clump and/or float to the top of the solution in which it is mixed.[36] To reduce this phenomenon, a reservoir syringe is connected to a 3-way stopcock and 3-mL syringe (**Fig. 18**). Using the connection between the 2 syringes, the particles can be agitated to maintain the proper suspension of the PVA.[1,34]

There are 2 keys to proper deployment of the PVA particles. One is injecting the particles with a smaller-size syringe to optimize control in the administration of the agent through the microcatheter and to minimize particle clumping, which can cause catheter occlusion (**Fig. 19**). The second key is the use of fluoroscopy to allow the IR to observe the administration of the particles in real time. The IR must be careful to ensure that no reflux of the material enters any nontarget vessels.[1,36] Once the blood

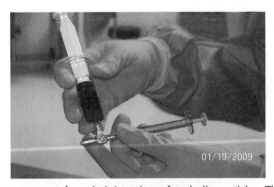

01/19/2009

**Fig. 18.** Syringe arrangement for administration of embolic particles. The 10-mL reservoir syringe (made of glass) contains beads, chemotherapy, contrast, and ethiodized oil. The metal stopcock prevents degradation. Attached to the stopcock is a 1-mL syringe (also glass) for agitating the mixture to ensure suspension and for controlled administration of the mixture.

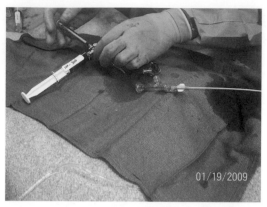

**Fig. 19.** Chemotherapy being administered via a microcatheter into a distal vessel branch for treatment of vascular tumor.

flow slows down, the particles are gently flushed out of the catheter and contrast is injected to confirm that the desired embolization result has been obtained. Additional embolization is performed in a gradual, stepwise fashion as needed, to ensure optimum results while minimizing the chance for nontarget embolization.

A calibrated form of PVA spheres (Contour SE Microspheres; Boston Scientific, Natick, MA, USA) is now available. Microspheres are constructed with a hydrophilic coating, which decreases the surface friction and minimizes clumping of the particles to reduce the chance of catheter occlusion. In theory, the use of PVA spheres also improves targeted embolization because of the ability of the spherical shape to more accurately occlude specific diameter vessels[39] and compressibility, which allows larger size particles to squeeze through smaller lumen microcatheters and out into smaller arterial branches (**Fig. 20**). Microspheres are packaged in a prefilled syringe, reducing the phenomenon of particles being left in the vial so that more complete use of the product can be accomplished. There is a question as to whether data support the benefits of Microspheres over traditional PVA particles.

In April 2000, the Food and Drug Administration (FDA) approved the use of Embosphere Microspheres (BioSphere Medical, Inc, Rockland, MA, USA) for use with

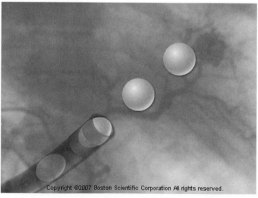

**Fig. 20.** Contour SE Microspheres. (*Courtesy of* Boston Scientific, Inc, Natick, MA, USA; with permission.)

hypervascularized tumors (ie, uterine fibroids) and arteriovenous malformations (**Fig. 21**) (http://www.biospheremed.com). Embospheres are synthetic, gelatin-coated, acrylic microspheres that are nonallergic and induce much less of an inflammatory response in vivo when compared with PVA embolization for treatment of fibroids (**Fig. 22**). There are 3 characteristics that allow Embospheres to be effective particulate agents (**Fig. 23**): (1) the agent is somewhat compressible, allowing it to be delivered easier via a microcatheter (**Fig. 24**); (2) each sphere has a hydrophilic coating, allowing smoother deployment with less particulate aggregation and more consistent suspension within a contrast solution; and (3) spheres are accurately calibrated to facilitate a more precise level of vessel occlusion. Embospheres are packaged in sterile prefilled syringes of spheres and saline. The spheres range in size from 100 to 1200 μm. After 8 mL of a specific contrast agent (nonionic, nonisosmolar contrast with 300 mg/mL iodine content) is added to the prefilled syringes, full and symmetric suspension of the Embospheres will take place within 20 minutes.

In 2001, the manufacturer placed a coating on the spheres, increasing the ability to visualize the microspheres in their packaging syringe ex vivo. This coating was called EmboGold (BioSphere Medical, Inc, Rockland, MA, USA; http://www.biospheremed.com). However, this product has been removed from the market because patients were shown to have a variety of reactions to this product, including more pain and systemic symptoms after uterine artery embolization.

Earlier this year the FDA approved a new particulate agent called Embozene Microsphere (CeloNova BioSciences, Inc, Newnan, GA, USA). This microsphere has a hydrogel core and is coated with a proprietary, synthetic, inorganic polymer called Polyzene-F (http://www.celanova.com) that renders Embozene extremely biocompatible and hemocompatible. Furthermore, the Polyzene-F coating is anti-inflammatory and resistant to bacteria. Embozene absorbs certain medications, raising the possibility of using this embolic for drug delivery to a target site. To increase visualization of the particles, each sphere size is manufactured with a dedicated color. Embozene Microspheres range from 40 to 1300 μm in diameter and are packaged in either vials or syringes with 1 to 2 mL of material (http://www.celanova.com). They are calibrated in size by 50-μm increments, increasing accuracy of the size of vessel embolized. Finally, like other synthetic microspheres on the market, Embozene spheres are compressible

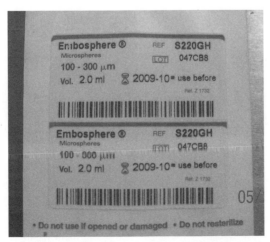

**Fig. 21.** Embospheres package. Marketed by Biosphere Medical, Inc, Rockland, MA, USA.

without fracturing or deforming (http://www.celanova.com). Along these lines are LC Beads (**Fig. 25**) (manufactured by Biocompatibles, Farnham, Surrey, UK [http://www.biocompatibles.com], distributed by AngioDynamics, Queensbury, NY, [http://www.angiodynamics.com]). These beads are created with a sulfonate-modified

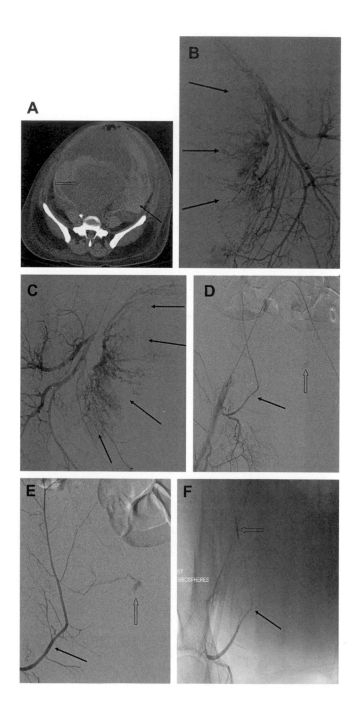

hydrogel that creates a negative charge, allowing binding of certain chemotherapeutic agents such as doxorubicin. The beads can then be deployed into the vessel feeding the tumor using superselective angiography. The beads provide controlled drug release over up to 14 days while also occluding distal blood flow to hypervascular tumor (http://www.biocompatibles.com).[40]

### Liquid agents

The first-line treatment for femoral pseudoaneurysms that occur after femoral artery catheterization is manual compression using ultrasound guidance.[41] If this maneuver fails, direct injection of thrombin (Thrombin-JMI; King Pharmaceuticals, Inc, Bristol, TN, USA) has been proven to be safe and successful.[41,42] Color flow and Doppler ultrasound guidance document the diameter and length of the neck of the pseudoaneurysm and monitor the flow in the pseudoaneurysm during the thrombin injection. The patient and ultrasound machine are sterilely prepped and draped. The access site is anesthetized with 1% lidocaine (10 mg/ml) buffered with sodium bicarbonate 8.4% (1 mEq/ml). The thrombin is reconstituted (**Fig. 26**) in solution to a concentration of 1000 units thrombin/mL. The pseudoaneurysm is accessed using a 25-gauge 3-cm long needle or a 22-gauge spinal needle, and is injected under color flow ultrasound observation. Care must be taken not to reflux thrombin into the normal vasculature. After complete thrombosis of the pseudoaneurysm is documented, the needle is removed, the access site is cleaned and bandaged, and the patient remains on bed rest for 4 to 6 hours.[41] Thrombin is also used to soak embolization coils before their deployment to quicken vessel thrombosis and decrease procedure time[33] as well as to thrombose aneurysms elsewhere in the body.[25]

Other liquid embolic agents include the class of sclerosing agents: absolute alcohol (Dehydrated Alcohol, Luitpold Pharmaceuticals, Inc, Shirley, NY, USA) (**Fig. 27**) and sodium tetradecyl sulfate (Sotradecol, AngioDynamics, Queensbury, NY, USA) (**Fig. 28**).

Absolute alcohol has been used intravascularly as an embolic agent for many years. One application has been the devascularization of renal cell carcinoma before surgery.[33] Absolute alcohol is also used in treatment of vascular malformations.[15–17]

◄━━━━━━━━━━━━━━━━━━━━━━━━━━━━━━━━━━━━━━━━━━━━

**Fig. 22.** Case study 2. A 27-year-old woman 2 days postpartum with healthy twins delivered via cesarean section. The patient subsequently developed HELLP syndrome (Hemolysis, Elevated Liver enzymes, Low Platelet count) with hepatic and renal failure. Angiography after unenhanced CT showed a large quantity of blood in the pelvis with extension to the abdomen, without a clear cause. After an extensive search in the patient's abdomen and pelvis, the source was ultimately identified in a medial branch of the right inferior epigastric artery, likely related to her incision. This was successfully embolized with 500- to 700-μm embospheres. (A) Axial CT scan shows high-density blood (*solid arrow*) throughout pelvis and surrounding postgravid uterus (*open arrow*). (B, C) Selective angiogram in the left and right internal iliac arteries. Normal vasculature of the uterus (*solid arrows*) without evidence of bleeding. (D) Selective angiogram of the right external iliac artery shows faint extravasation over the midpelvis (*open arrow*), thought to originate from the right inferior epigastric artery (*solid arrow*). (E) Selective angiogram of the right inferior epigastric artery (*solid arrow*) confirms extravasation from small medial branch of the vessel (*open arrow*). (F) Postembolization angiogram after infusion of 500- to 700-μm embospheres. Microcoils were placed distally in the right inferior epigastric artery (*open arrow*) before embospheres to protect distal branches from embolization. Note stagnant contrast in the inferior epigastric artery after embolization (*solid arrow*) with no evidence of extravasation.

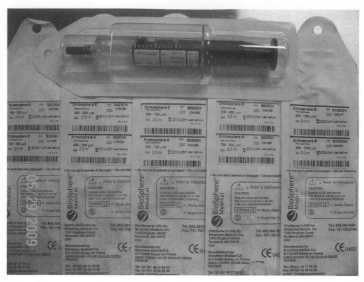

**Fig. 23.** Embospheres come in multiple sizes. The packages are color coded to aid in identification. Size ranges from 100 to 1200 μm.

Absolute alcohol works on the endothelial lining of the vessel, denaturing protein in the cell wall and causing cell death by dehydration and leading to thrombus.[36] Because of its liquid nature, alcohol can penetrate to the arteriole and capillary level.[1,34] Treatment of vascular malformations requires an experienced operator and close observation because of the permanent tissue or nerve injury that can occur with extravasation of alcohol or the occlusion of small end arteries.[34,36] When delivered intra-arterially, an occlusion balloon or a blood pressure (BP) cuff is used to prevent reflux of the material into the normal vasculature and minimize the flow of alcohol into the systemic circulation.[16,33,43] Injection of alcohol intravascularly can be painful, so the patient should be well sedated or, in the case of a vascular malformation, asleep under general anesthesia.[15]

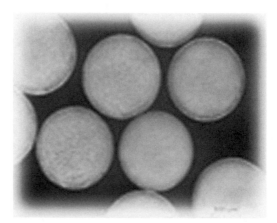

**Fig. 24.** Embozene Microspheres designed by CeloNova BioSciences, Inc, Newnan, GA, USA.

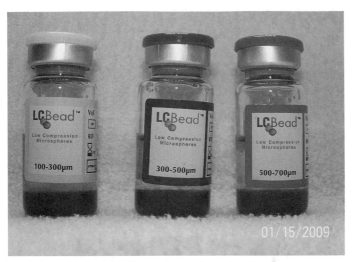

**Fig. 25.** LC beads in multiple sizes. Note color coding of packages.

The volume of alcohol injected is predetermined by the volume of contrast needed to fill the appropriate vascular branches through the catheter with the balloon inflated. The alcohol is injected through the catheter with the balloon inflated and a timer is started. Some IRs infuse 100 mg of lidocaine intra-arterially before injecting the alcohol to minimize the pain associated with this procedure. After approximately 5 minutes, the catheter is aspirated to remove any alcohol that may be floating in the vessel. The occlusion balloon is then deflated. Contrast is infused to assess for

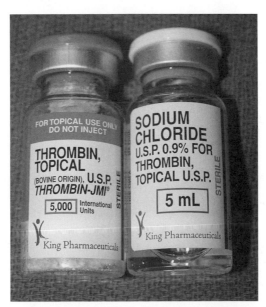

**Fig. 26.** Thrombin in vial; comes as a powder with premeasured sterile 0.9% sodium chloride as diluent.

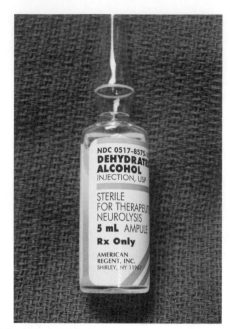

**Fig. 27.** Absolute or dehydrated alcohol.

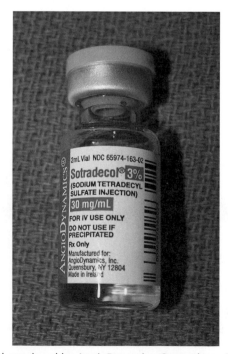

**Fig. 28.** Sotradecol vial, produced by AngioDynamics, Queensbury, NY, USA.

vascular occlusion. If any other feeding vessels remain patent, the process is repeated.[16,17,44]

An alternative liquid sclerosing agent that is used for embolization procedures is sodium tetradecyl sulfate (STS) (Sotradecol; AngioDynamics, Inc, Queensbury, NY, USA). Sotradecol is more forgiving to the surrounding tissue than absolute alcohol and is likely to be used for venous malformations, especially those close to nerves or the skin surface and small (<3 mm) varicose veins (pelvic, legs, gastric).[45–47] Sotradecol is manufactured in 1% and 3% solutions, available in 2-mL vials. The size of the malformation and its proximity to the skin surface and nerves determine the strength of solution used; the 3% solution is generally used for larger malformations, gastric and pelvic varicosities. Use of more than 20 mL in a single setting should be done with caution. Sotradecol is a saponification agent, and when mixed with air creates a foam.[47] The theoretical advantage of STS foam is that the STS, with surfactant on the surface of each bubble, comes into better contact with the vessel wall, displacing the liquid volume of blood or lymph,[46] allowing embolization of larger vessels than solution alone.[48] The theoretical risk of using STS foam is that when the air comes out of solution, the air can embolize to the heart. In most cases, small amounts of air embolizing to the heart is not an issue but can be problematic if the patient has a patent foramen ovale.[46]

The first generation of a rapidly hardening plastic adhesive that was chemically similar to "Superglue" was isobutyl 2-cyanoacrylate (Ethicon, Inc, Somerville, NJ, USA).[35] Historically, this adhesive has been used medically since the 1960s, but was not used in radiology until the 1970s. Because of its documented carcinogenic effects in animals, this formulation is used only experimentally in the United States. However, a second-generation glue, N-butyl-2-cyanoacrylate (TRUFILL n-BCA; Cordis Neurovascular, Inc, Miami Lakes, FL, USA) has gained wide usage in the United States (**Fig. 29**). Both glues polymerize (link molecules to form a strong bond) when they come in contact with ionic solutions (blood) and the epithelium. These products should only be handled by experienced operators who know the characteristics of these acrylates.

n-BCA is packaged with tantalum powder and an ethiodized oil-based contrast agent (Ethiodol; Nycomed US, Inc, Melville, NY, USA) (**Fig. 30**). The tantalum powder provides fluoroscopic radiopacity to the material, whereas Ethiodol increases the

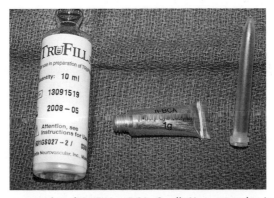

**Fig. 29.** N-Butyl-2-cyanoacrylate (TRUFILL n-BCA, Cordis Neurovascular, Inc, Miami Lakes, FL, USA).

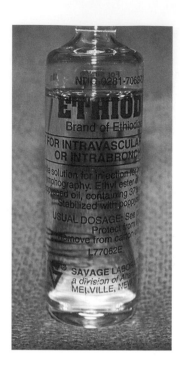

**Fig. 30.** Ethiodol in vial.

polymerization time. The polymerization time is determined according to the target of embolotherapy.

Arterial-venous malformations (AVM) are the main indication for n-BCA. However, applications have expanded to include other pathologies ranging from type II endoleaks to portal vein embolization. Each type of embolization requires a different polymerization time. The ratio between Ethiodol and glue increases, varying from 3:1 to 8:1, because more time is needed to disperse the polymer throughout the vasculature. Thus, AVMs require a fast setting time, and use less ethiodol than a right portal vein embolization, which requires more glue volume to occlude the different branches of the vessel.[11,43,49]

Glue is administered through a guided coaxial system (a catheter or sheath with a longer catheter inside it, allowing rapid removal of the internal catheter without loss of access). This system can be either a guiding sheath/catheter combination, or a catheter/microcatheter system. After placing the guiding sheath/catheter into position, a microcatheter or diagnostic catheter is manipulated through the existing catheter and out distally to the area being embolized. As with all embolic agents, glue is mixed on a separate table using a glass shot glass. Dextrose infusion is performed before n-BCA administration to prevent ionic solutions in the catheter from initiating the polymerization process prematurely. The catheter or microcatheter is pulled after the volume of glue is injected and before the adhesive can harden and adhere the catheter to the vessel.[34] Accidental adherence of the catheter within the glue polymer is one of the biggest concerns with administration of n-BCA.[49]

In 2005, the FDA approved the use of the liquid embolic agent ethylene vinyl alcohol (Onyx LES, ev3 Endovascular, Inc, Minneapolis, MN, USA) for use with cerebral vascular malformations (**Fig. 31**). Onyx is a nonadhesive copolymer that is composed

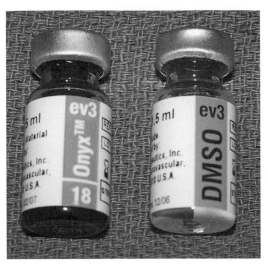

**Fig. 31.** Onyx in package before administration.

of ethylene vinyl alcohol (EVOH) and tantalum powder (mentioned earlier), and dissolved in a solvent agent dimethyl sulfoxide (DMSO) (http://www.fda.gov). Onyx solid-
ifies when it comes in contact with blood or other liquid agents (normal saline, water).[50]
Cyanoacrylate (n-BCA) must be delivered fairly rapidly via the catheter, followed by
immediate retrieval of the catheter to prevent it from being glued to the artery. Onyx
is injected gradually, more like caulking or toothpaste (**Fig. 32**). Injection of Onyx
may occur over a 10- to 30-minute time interval, gradually pushing the material into
the nidus of the target lesion. Unlike cyanoacrylate, it is rare for the catheter to become
permanently glued to the vessel. The catheter can become adhered to the Onyx, but
gradual and continuous traction on the catheter over a period of several minutes
usually results in successful removal of the microcatheter.[34]

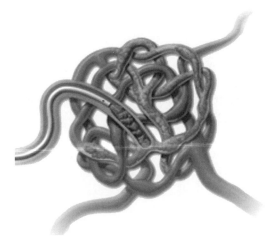

**Fig. 32.** Schematic diagram of Onyx injected into vessels.

The original product line of Onyx consisted of 2 types: Onyx 18 that contains 6% EVOH, and Onyx 34 that contains 8% EVOH. Onyx 18 has a lower viscosity, which allows it to have greater penetration into the nidus of the AVM than Onyx 34. However, in high-flow malformations or fistulas, the higher viscous Onyx 34 is suggested to minimize nontarget embolization of the venous circulation and ultimately the lungs.[50] In 2007, ev3 received FDA approval for a new product line, Onyx HD 500, which is 20% EVOH and indicated for the treatment of intracranial aneurysms (http://www.medicalnewstoday.com) (ev3 Endovascular, Inc, Plymouth, MN, USA).

Case study 3. Onyx was used to seal an endoleak postabdominal aortic stent graft. An abdominal aortic stent graft was placed in a patient. Follow-up imaging demonstrated continued filling of the aneurysmal sac, despite adequate seal of the stent graft. Angiography revealed a branch of the inferior colic artery feeding the sac. This branch was accessed using a microcatheter and embolized using Onyx (**Figs. 33** and **34**).

Products necessary for administration of Onyx include a DMSO-compatible microcatheter and the Onyx mechanical shaker. The ev3 microcatheters (Echelon, Rebar, and Marathon) are all DMSO compatible. Other manufacturers have also developed microcatheters that are DMSO compatible. Onyx is packaged in a kit with 1.5 mL Onyx, 1.5 mL DMSO, and syringes compatible for use with these solutions. The Onyx mechanical shaker holds up to 4 vials of Onyx. Onyx should be shaken for 20 minutes before use.[50] Setting "8" allows for proper mixing of the tantalum for best visualization of Onyx during fluoroscopy.

Once the location of the microcatheter has been confirmed, DMSO is injected using the DMSO syringe before administration of the Onyx. The hub of the catheter and DMSO syringe are held upright (vertically), and the dead space in the hub is filled with the remaining DMSO in the syringe to prevent air embolism. The Onyx is drawn up in the Onyx-labeled syringe with an 18-gauge needle and connected to the

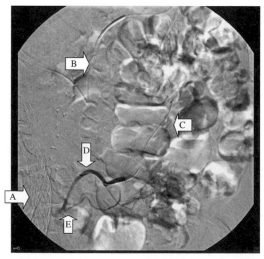

**Fig. 33.** Accessing the leak using microcatheter technology. (A) The stent graft in vivo. (B) A 5F catheter used to access the superior mesenteric artery. (C) Microcatheter through regular catheter passes through left and inferior colic to the IMA. (D) Catheter tip in the inferior mesenteric artery. (E) Aneurysm sac continuing to fill with blood, fed by the inferior mesenteric artery.

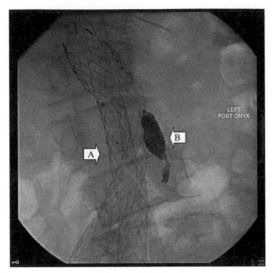

**Fig. 34.** Image of aneurysm post treatment. (A) Endovascular stent visible. (B) Onyx ball filling aneurysm sac and blocking feeder vessel.

microcatheter in a wet-to-wet technique. Onyx is slowly injected to clear the DMSO, which if injected too fast can cause vasospasm and/or angionecrosis. It should then be infused at a recommended rate of (0.16 mL/min), not to exceed 0.3 mL/min.[51] If Onyx is given too fast and refluxes more than 1 cm from the tip of the microcatheter, the microcatheter may become lodged in the Onyx. Onyx begins to create a skinlike film once injected into the body, and complete solidification occurs within 5 minutes.[50] Thus, it is important that little time is wasted during the transition between multiple syringes. If the operator feels resistance in the microcatheter the injection should be stopped, and the catheter system evaluated and replaced if necessary. To remove the microcatheter after the Onyx injection, it is recommended to wait a few seconds and then aspirate the contents of the microcatheter, followed by gently pulling the microcatheter out of the Onyx cast.

## APPLICATIONS

The improvements in the ability to safely catheterize and embolize specific vessels have led to a variety of uses for embolotherapy. The following sections are by no means a complete list of uses for this procedure but rather an overview of applications of this technology.

### *Control of Bleeding*

The ability to embolize vessels ruptured or damaged as a result of trauma, tumor ingrowth, and inflammatory or ulcerative diseases reduces the need for surgery and can help to improve patient outcomes. In many cases of life-threatening trauma and associated refractory bleeding, surgical fixation of fractures is followed by embolization of the bleeding vessels or vice versa to decrease morbidity and mortality and reduce transfusion needs.[8] Pelvic, extremity, vertebral body, hepatic, renal, and splenic artery injuries, and many other arterial injuries can be effectively treated with embolotherapy.[2–6,8] Emergent hysterectomy was once the only option for severe postpartum hemorrhage.[37] The ability to embolize uterine arteries with Gelfoam allows the opportunity for immediate control of hemorrhage, with the benefit of later vessel recanalization and salvage of the uterus and child-bearing capabilities.[9]

Gastrointestinal (GI) bleeding from an arterial source has effectively been treated by embolization.[3,4] When endoscopic therapy is ineffective or cannot be performed because of excessive blood in the GI tract, angiography may not only pinpoint caus-ative source of bleeding but may also allow definitive treatment.[3] This procedure requires the patient to be actively bleeding at the time contrast is injected to show contrast extravasation from the bleeding vessel. Ability to embolize within the GI tract is also dependent on the ability to occlude blood flow through a particular vessel without causing nontargeted bowel ischemia. Collateral circulation to the upper GI tract is fairly robust, so embolotherapy has been widely used to treat Mallory-Weiss tears, hemorrhagic gastritis, hemobilia, and hemosuccus pancreaticus (bleeding from the pancreas) with low risk for causing end-organ infarction.[4] However, with the lower GI tract (small bowel and colon), collateral flow is less prominent and embo-lotherapy is associated with a higher risk for bowel infarction. With improvements in microcatheter and microcoil technology, superselective target embolization has been enhanced. However, care must still be taken to avoid embolizing vessels that may cause infarction of the small bowel or the colon; thus empiric embolization of small bowel or colonic vessels is not recommended.[4] Because GI bleeding is typically intermittent, the ability to identify the source of bleeding angiographically can be frus-trating, with angiography showing the bleeding source in fewer than 40% of cases.[4] Therefore, a patient may be actively bleeding on the nursing unit but not at the exact time of the angiographic procedure. Endoscopic control of GI bleeding remains the first-line therapy.[3]

GI bleeding from a venous source is usually related to portal hypertension or splenic vein thrombosis causing variceal hemorrhaging.[52] If endoscopy fails to control the source of bleeding, transcatheter techniques have been used.[23,25,52] With bleeding due to portal hypertension, a transjugular intrahepatic portosystemic shunt (TIPS) can be created to reduce portal pressures and stop the bleeding. If a TIPS does not control the bleeding, direct catheterization of the varices via the TIPS can be per-formed, followed by embolization with a liquid sclerosant and coils or AVP to control the bleeding.[53] Balloon retrograde transvenous obliteration of the varices using Sotra-decol foam can also be done on an elective basis to treat intermittently bleeding gastric varices related to portal hypertension, splenic vein thrombosis, or large sple-norenal shunt causing left-sided portal hypertension.[54,55]

Bronchial artery embolization (BAE) is used to control recurrent or massive hemop-tysis in patients with chronic inflammatory lung diseases, tuberculosis, and bronchio-genic cancers.[2,6] BAE can be performed emergently or nonemergently, and requires a detailed knowledge of bronchial arterial anatomy and additional possible sources of collateral bleeding, such as the phrenic artery or intercostal arteries.[2] BAE is commonly performed using PVA particles. Whenever possible, the use of coils is avoided because recurrence of bleeding may occur, especially with chronic inflamma-tory processes.[2]

On rare occasions, hemoptysis may be caused by bleeding from the pulmonary artery. Trauma due to pulmonary artery catheters, mycotic aneurysms due to tubercu-losis, or pulmonary AVMs as seen with Osler-Weber-Rendu disease are common causes. Embolization is usually performed with a variety of occlusive agents such as coils or AVPs.[32,56]

Neurologic emergencies resulting from hemorrhage may respond to embolization. The source of hemorrhage may be vascular malformations, aneurysm rupture, refrac-tory epistaxis, or traumatic injury. Each cause for the bleeding is handled differently, and the agents used are tailored to the specific source for bleeding.[43,57,58] On occasion, preoperative embolization of brain or nerve sheath tumors is performed, typically with the use of PVA.

### Controlling Pain or Other Symptoms

Vascular malformations are congenital abnormalities of blood vessels that result in the presence of too many vessels and can involve the lymphatics, veins, and arteries. When there is an abnormal communication between the arteries and veins it is called an arteriovenous malformation or AVM. These vascular malformations develop in utero and are classified according to structure, location, and natural progression of the malformation. The malformations are often categorized as either high-flow or low-flow, depending on whether there is an abnormal communication between the artery and vein (high-flow) or if the abnormal vessels primarily involve the veins and/ or the lymphatics (low-flow).

Although some vascular malformations are diagnosed and treated in childhood, many of them remain asymptomatic and undiagnosed until adulthood.[15] High-flow vascular malformations can cause a variety of symptoms, depending on their size and location. When located in cerebral vasculature, rupture of these malformations can be devastating.[57] When located in the lungs, hypoxemia and paradoxic cerebral emboli can occur.[19] When in an extremity, steal of flow from more peripheral tissue can lead to symptomatic ischemia.[17] If the arterial to venous communications are large, high-output cardiac failure can result.[46] When possible, catheter-directed or direct puncture embolotherapy with agents that obliterate the nidus of the vascular malformation is the treatment of choice. Absolute alcohol, Sotradecol, cyanoacrylate, Onyx, and particulate agents have all been used by themselves or in combination with other agents.[16,46,49,59]

Low-flow vascular malformations can also occur anywhere in the body and can be any size. Venous malformations (VMs) are composed primarily of veins, but can be mixed and involve capillary and lymphatic vessels. VMs are less prone to hemorrhage but can be a significant cause of pain and disability. Treatment involves embolization of the VM with absolute alcohol or STS used as a foam or pure liquid agent. Patients often require multiple treatment sessions and need lifetime follow-up. Treatment is most often palliative, and is geared toward minimizing symptoms and trying to obliterate as much of the malformation as possible; it is rarely curative. Vascular malformations seem to grow during growth spurts, with hormonal stimulation (puberty, pregnancy, and birth control pills), and after trauma (including surgery).[15,16,46]

The advancement in technology surrounding endovascular repair of thoracic and abdominal aortic aneurysms combined with advances in embolotherapy techniques have allowed for intravascular treatment of aortic aneurysms and some of their associated complications, such as endoleaks.[39] Embolization is used before endovascular aneurysm repair (EVAR) to treat arterial branches that communicate with the aneurysm and may cause retrograde flow, creating an endoleak after EVAR.[60] Vessels embolized before EVAR include the hypogastric, inferior mesenteric, accessory renal, celiac, superior mesenteric, and the subclavian arteries.[39] Embolization is also used after EVAR to treat endoleaks (blood flow that occurs within the aneurysm sac after endograft repair).[61,62] Endoleak repair can be done percutaneously or intravascularly, depending on the type and location of the endoleaks.

The emergent use of uterine artery embolization (UAE) for postpartum bleeding has been previously discussed. Another application of UAE is the treatment of uterine fibroids. This condition affects 20% to 40% of women, usually aged 35 years and older.[9]

Uterine fibroids are symptomatic in 10% to 20% of women and are associated with excessive bleeding, pain, pressure, heaviness, constipation, and painful intercourse.[7] Microsphere or PVA particles are used to obstruct blood flow to the fibroids, significantly reducing symptoms in 85% to 90% of cases.[9]

Gonadal vein embolization has been used for treatment of valvular incompetence of the gonadal vein associated with symptomatic varicoceles in men for more than 20 years.[18] Men with varicoceles often present with oligospermia or abnormal sperm motility, and pain in the scrotal area due to the varicose veins around the testicle. Analogous to varicoceles in men, women can develop painful pelvic varices secondary to valvular incompetence of the gonadal vein, and have shown improvement after gonadal vein embolization. In both men and women the pain can be debilitating, but because of the complex differential diagnosis associated with pelvic pain in women versus scrotal pain for men, pelvic varices as a cause for pelvic pain in women is underdiagnosed and many times missed altogether.[63]

Palliative treatment of many cancers can involve transcatheter embolization to relieve pain or in preparation for palliative surgery (ie, metal rod for a pathologic fracture at the site of a metastatic bone lesion). Bony metastases often respond to embolization, which does not eliminate the tumor but reduces the blood flow, alleviating pain and also making it less likely that the patient will have significant bleeding with placement of an orthopedic device (ie, rod).[29]

### Embolization for the Treatment of Malignant Tumors

The role of catheter-directed embolization in the treatment of hypervascular malignant tumors has gained wider acceptance in the past 15 years, especially for cases in which the liver is involved. Hepatocellular carcinoma (HCC) is a primary liver cancer, often arising from diseased liver cells in cirrhotic patients or patients with a prior history of viral hepatitis (hepatitis B or C). These tumors derive more than 95% of their blood flow from the hepatic artery, whereas the liver itself derives most of its blood flow from the portal vein (75%), with the hepatic artery contributing 25% of the flow.[26] In situations where the portal vein is patent and liver function is adequate, segments of the hepatic artery can be embolized, depriving these tumors of their blood flow and therefore their primary food and oxygen supply.[26] At many institutions, transarterial chemoembolization (TACE) is performed using a combination of particulate matter and one or more chemotherapeutic agents mixed with iodized oil (Ethiodol; Nycomed US, Inc, Melville, NY, USA).[10] Ethiodol tends to accumulate within the malignant cells and carries the chemotherapeutic agents with it. The principle with TACE is to obstruct arterial inflow to the tumor, while the adjacent normal liver and bile duct cells continue to receive their nutrition via the portal venous system. Malignant cells that remain viable are then in an environment with high local concentrations of chemotherapeutic drugs (ie, doxorubicin), which is designed to kill the growing malignant cells that survive the ischemic insult from the particulate embolization. Originally used exclusively with HCC (or primary liver cancer), TACE is gaining acceptance for use with a wide variety of liver metastases.[10,11,13] In these situations, systemic chemotherapy and surgical resection remain front-line therapies, with TACE being used when the metastatic disease is primarily in the liver, and is no longer responding to systemic chemotherapy or is inoperable.[27,28,44] In the case of metastatic carcinoid, embolization is recommended when symptoms cannot be managed with octreotide therapy (Sandostatin LAR; Novartis Pharmaceuticals, Cambridge, MA, USA) or when the volume of tumor burden reaches 50% of the liver volume.[10,64] A new therapy being investigated in the treatment of primary renal and liver cancer involves the use of small, low-compression hydrogel microspheres in sizes of 100 to 300, 300 to 500, or 500 to

700 µm (Biocompatibles International, Farnham, Surrey, UK), immersed in a mixture of either doxorubicin (for liver cancer) or irinotecan (for renal cell cancer). These drug-carrying microspheres are then used to perform the embolization. Patients usually require between 1 and 3 embolization sessions, repeated as needed. Systemic side effects of this treatment are fewer than those of traditional TACE.[40,65]

Angiomyolipomas are benign neoplasms consisting primarily of fat, smooth muscle, and vascular components. Angiomyolipomas are usually located in the kidney, affecting 0.3% to 3% of the population and more prevalent in patients with tuberous sclerosis complex.[66] The average age of onset is 43 years, and 40% of tumors are symptomatic. Aside from discomfort caused by tumor bulk, there is a risk of hemorrhage from the vascular components of the tumor. Embolization of the tumor is performed to treat bulk symptoms and bleeding; it is indicated for tumors greater than 4 cm in diameter to reduce the risk of hemorrhage.[66]

### Reducing Blood Loss During Surgery

Presurgical embolization is an effective tool to aid in minimizing blood loss at the time of surgery. Targets of presurgical embolotherapy include the kidney, uterus, pancreas, brain, neck, mediastinum, posterior thorax, extremity, and pelvis.[20,24,25] The patient arrives in the IR suite on the day of surgery, where liquid agents, coils, and particles are used in an individually tailored fashion to obstruct blood flow to the intended target.[30] The patient is placed on either a patient-controlled analgesic pump immediately post procedure, or epidural anesthesia for pain control if necessary until surgery can be performed. In cases in which the embolization is not associated with too much pain, it can performed 48 hours to several weeks before surgery, depending on whether simple cessation of blood flow or tumor shrinkage is the goal.[25]

Embolization of the portal vein is performed in patients with marginal liver reserve before planned resection of that lobe or segment of the liver. For example, embolization of the right portal vein encourages hypertrophy of the left lobe of the liver in preparation for right lobe resection. The degree of liver hypertrophy experienced after embolization is directly related to the volume of liver embolized (from as little as 2.4% with subsegmental embolization, to 46% increase in the left lobe after right portal vein embolization).[20]

The patient receives a follow-up computed tomography (CT) or MR imaging scan 30 days after embolization, and is scheduled for surgery if sufficient hypertrophy has developed.[20,22]

Treatment of arterial and/or venous collaterals before a Fontan procedure or cavopulmonary anastomosis surgery helps to improve success of the surgical procedure. In addition, these patients are evaluated periodically after surgery for development of collaterals, which are then embolized.[56]

The previously described clinical scenarios represent a few of the multiple applications of embolization procedures routinely performed at the authors' institution. Using an array of embolic materials and techniques, virtually any hypervascular area that could cause hemorrhage or cause symptoms can be treated using embolotherapy techniques.

### NURSING CARE AND EMBOLIZATION PROCEDURES
#### Preparing a Patient for an Embolization Procedure

Patients should be seen and evaluated by the interventional radiology team before any procedure. For elective cases, a patient may be seen in the outpatient clinic where the following issues can be addressed: the indications for the procedure based on a good history and review of prior treatments, imaging, and laboratory data; a thorough discussion of potential risks, benefits, and alternatives to the planned procedure; allergies and current medications; specific history of coagulopathies or current anticoagulation use; medical history of back or other difficulties that would impact the patient's ability to lie on a procedure table for several hours; respiratory and cardiac issues that would affect sedation/analgesia and fluid and oxygen management; renal function and dietary issues; functional reserve; overall prognosis; and transportation and home care related issues. Recent imaging is essential to allow for optimum planning of the procedure. In the case of UAE, it is important to determine that the excessive bleeding is in fact due to leiomyomatosis and not a malignancy or some other etiological factor.[7] Cancer patients need recent (<3 months) imaging to verify the size and location of tumor and evaluate for metastatic disease. Candidates for TACE must have satisfactory liver reserve, and those candidates for portal vein embolization must have intact arterial and portal flow to the target growth area, without tumor invasion.[22] Patients with vascular malformations require current MR imaging to evaluate and localize the malformation.[16]

As IR procedures require the use of iodinated contrast material, awareness of renal function is essential (**Fig. 35**). A serum creatinine level below 1.5 mg/dL is preferable, with an estimated glomerular filtration rate greater than 50 mL/min.[67] Vitamin C, N-acetylcysteine, and sodium bicarbonate infusion can all be administered preprocedurally in patients with compromised renal function in an effort to reduce the risk for contrast-induced nephropathy (CIN).[68–70] Other measures that are used to minimize the risk for CIN include diluting the contrast material, minimizing the volume of contrast used, and using carbon dioxide ($CO_2$) gas as a contrast medium.[67] Emergent cases require a risk/benefit analysis of potential renal side effects versus the risk of not performing the procedure. Often, the embolization procedure can be life saving but

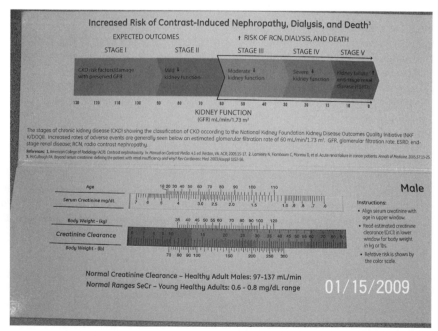

**Fig. 35.** Slide rule produced by Visipaque, which estimates a patient's risk for contrast-induced nephropathy based on age, sex, weight, and serum creatinine level.

creates a secondary renal problem that in the worst-case scenario would require either transient or long-term dialysis therapy.

Hematological disorders do not preclude the performance of an embolization procedure but require special preparation and planning to manage the bleeding risks safely. The preferred international normalized ratio (INR) for arterial punctures is less than 1.5 and for venous punctures less than 2.0.[68] Patients on therapeutic oral warfarin either need to stop it for 4 days or be transitioned to a shorter-acting drug, such as a low molecular weight heparin, before the procedure. Those with a physiologically high INR may require vitamin K or fresh frozen plasma preprocedure, and in some cases the patient may need to be admitted the night before for medical management. Patients with hemophilia need a hematology consult because they need to be treated with the appropriate infusions of specific factors in the periprocedural period. The effectiveness of any embolization procedure may be reduced in patients with a coagulopathy, because all embolic agents depend on the ability of the body to mount a thrombotic response when flow in a vessel is decreased. Acetylsalicylic acid (aspirin) and clopidogrel (Plavix; Bristol Meyers Squibb, New York, NY, USA) are often not routinely stopped before an embolization procedure, unless the patient is actively bleeding. Even in the presence of active bleeding, patients with a drug-eluting coronary stent should be evaluated by a cardiologist before stopping clopidogrel.[67,68]

Patients undergoing embolization of the spleen must receive immunizations before the procedure. The common recommended immunizations are *Streptococcus pneumoniae*, *Haemophilus influenzae* B, and *Neisseria meningitidis*. The immunizations should be administered about 14 days before the procedure to allow them to take effect in case total splenic infarction occurs. If it is not possible to provide the immunizations in advance, they should be administered as close to the time of the procedure as possible.[25] Most IRs also give these patients prophylactic antibiotics.[52]

An extensive evaluation is not always possible or practical in preparing for an emergent procedure, but certain preprocedure precautions should be undertaken. The INR must be normalized before or during the procedure. In many cases, normalization of the INR alone will stop bleeding and render the embolization procedure unnecessary.[4] A CT angiogram- or nuclear medicine-tagged red blood cell scan (red cells are withdrawn and tagged with a nuclear medicine particle, then reinjected, and the patient is moved to a nuclear medicine scanner to pinpoint the area of bleeding) may identify or localize the causative vessels or region that is bleeding.[3] Renal function must be evaluated. Some studies can be performed with $CO_2$ gas as a contrast medium in patients with impaired renal function. Careful technique is needed for $CO_2$ studies. In addition, $CO_2$ is contraindicated in the evaluation of arteries above the diaphragm because of the risk of neurologic complications.[4]

Liver function must be evaluated before any procedure affecting hepatic arterial or portal venous flow. Embolization can cause enough liver damage in patients with bilirubin levels greater than 2 mg/dL and marginal functional reserve to push them into liver failure. Patients with dilated or obstructed bile ducts are at higher risk for abscess formation and liver damage after TACE because blood flow to the bile ducts is primarily arterial.[27]

Immediately preprocedure, patients undergoing transarterial embolization are hydrated with 0.9% sodium chloride, usually at 150 to 200 mL/h. A steroid such as dexamethasone, 8 to 10 mg slow intravenous push, is given to reduce inflammation and nausea post embolization. H2 blockers (Famotidine; Merck & Co, Inc, Whitehouse Station, NJ, USA) and antihistamines (Benadryl; McNeil-PPC, Inc, Fort Washington, PA, USA) may also be given to reduce nausea associated with the embolization procedure. Prophylactic antibiotic therapy is standard, with the drugs used being broad-spectrum, but geared toward the types of organisms usually present in the region treated.[67,68,71] Most patients tolerate an embolization procedure with moderate (conscious) sedation. Patients undergoing UAE may also have epidural anesthesia begun before the procedure because ischemic pain can begin immediately after the procedure and be moderately severe. National and institutional policies on sedation are followed with all patients.[68]

### Intraprocedural Nursing Care

Although the specific vessels and target organ being treated may differ, the procedure itself is similar for any catheter-directed transarterial embolization. The femoral artery is accessed using the standard Seldinger technique. Rarely, the brachial artery (usually left) is accessed because of inability or inadvisability of using the femoral artery. In venous cases the femoral, jugular, or basilic vein is used. Angiography is used to map and study the vessels of concern. In cases of bleeding, extravasation of contrast is sought. The extravasation becomes visible as contrast from an intravascular location exits the bleeding vessel and accumulates at the site of bleeding. Microcatheters (3F or less) are often used to superselect (advance the catheter tip over a guidewire into a specific branch) specific vessels for evaluation and treatment (**Figs. 36** and **37**). Heparin is often administered intra-arterially to prevent thrombus formation in small vessels accessed with microcatheters. This part of the procedure is not painful. However, once embolization begins and areas are deprived of blood flow, ischemic pain may begin. Many physicians use ketorolac (Toradol; Roche Pharmaceuticals, Madison, WI, USA), 30 mg administered intravenously at this point, in addition to opioid analgesics such as fentanyl. Success of embolization is indicated by stagnation or lack of contrast flow within the target vessel(s).

During the procedure, the patient is under continuous nursing observation (**Fig. 38**). Heart rate, respiratory rate, BP, and oxygen saturation are documented every 5 minutes. The patient should receive continuous electrocardiographic and oxygen saturation monitoring. Low-flow oxygen is administered and adjusted to keep the oxygen level at or above 95%. Profound hypotension, bradycardia, or falling $O_2$

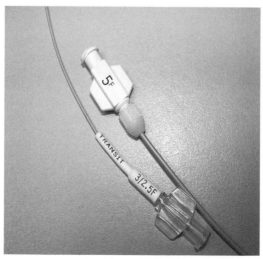

**Fig. 36.** A 5F catheter and a microcatheter used for embolization of small vessels, side by side.

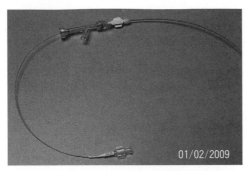

**Fig. 37.** The microcatheter is inserted into the catheter with a catheter control device connecting the two.

saturation levels are all indications to stop the case and assess the patient further. The nurse monitoring the patient must be comfortable in assessment and leadership skills because the nurse has the latitude to request a pause in the procedure to allow for further clinical evaluation of the patient. Conscious sedation protocols are used during the procedure, but the patient needs to be arousable in order to hold his or her breath as small vessels are being assessed.[68]

Embolization of VMs begins after the patient is placed under general anesthesia and the area of abnormality is prepped and draped in a sterile fashion.[15,49,51] If the malformation is in the extremity, sterile tourniquets may be placed to prevent the liquid embolic agent from passing through the normal outflow veins. The malformation is directly accessed using ultrasound guidance. Injection of nonionic contrast confirms an intraluminal needle location, and the venous anatomy is defined by injecting a measured volume of contrast.

Embolization is done with either alcohol or STS, followed by embolization of the needle tract with a Gelfoam slurry. Because of the nature of venous malformation there may be multiple pockets of abnormal veins, which may require multiple access sites into the malformation on order to perform the embolization. Although systemic side

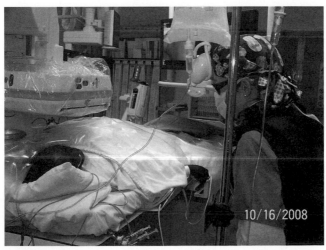

**Fig. 38.** Nursing assessment, close monitoring, and patient interaction are essential to a successful procedure.

effects are rare, they include hemolysis and, rarely, cardiac arrest. For this reason, anesthesia provides the necessary level of sedation for these procedures.

### Care of the Patient Following the Procedure

Assessment and interventions in the 24 hours post embolization are directed at managing pain, prevention of infection, and management of postembolization syndrome (PES). Frequent assessment during this period is essential. The patient is observed continuously for the first hour to discourage excessive movement that could cause the arterial access site to bleed or develop a hematoma.[68,71] Heart rate, BP, respiratory rate and character, oxygen saturation (SpO$_2$), and the access site are all monitored every 15 minutes in the early postprocedure period, as are the distal pulses if an arterial puncture is involved. (A risk of any arteriogram is the dislodgment of thrombus or atherosclerotic plaque, causing a distal embolus that obstructs blood flow to an extremity.)[72]

Pain is expected after embolization. Premedication is intended to reduce the inflammatory response associated with the PES. Some patients also suffer because of ischemic pain, depending on the target anatomy. Patient-controlled analgesia is started as soon as the procedure is completed to properly manage pain. Doses should be titrated to effect. Institutional policies for postprocedure pain control should be followed.

PES is an expected side effect of embolization.[73,74] The cause is unknown, but it is thought to be an inflammatory response to ischemia and necrosis.[75] PES begins immediately, peaks 24 to 48 hours post procedure, and can last up to 10 days. Symptoms include low-grade fever, nausea, vomiting, malaise, and generalized muscle aching, in addition to localized pain. The severity and duration varies for each patient; potential indicators of severity are under study.[73] Use of steroids and anti-inflammatory agents aid in the palliation of symptoms. Clear liquids are recommended for the first 12 hours post procedure to prevent nausea.

After 24 hours, most patients achieve manageable pain relief with oral analgesics and tolerate solid food. A fever of over 101°F (38.5°C) and/or intractable pain indicates abscess formation or sepsis, and requires ultrasound or CT imaging to evaluate. Careful attention to bowel motility is important. The use of opioids slows bowel motility, and the inflammatory process can cause pain, which is worsened by straining, resulting in severe constipation.[68]

## COMPLICATIONS OF EMBOLIZATION

Nontarget embolization with resulting ischemia is a risk of any embolization procedure. Symptoms vary from small areas of skin necrosis to loss of bowel, or ischemic damage to the brain or spinal cord or other end organs, depending on the location. Skill in technique and careful selection of vessels to be treated is the best prevention, although use of distal filters, occlusion balloons, and compression of venous drainage are all used with good effect.[1,8,15,21,25,43,61,76]

Leukocytosis post embolization is also found in some populations. The degree of leukocytosis does not directly correlate with symptoms of systemic infection and is thought to be a consequence of the inflammatory process associated with embolization. Careful assessment of clinical status along with laboratory evaluation is needed to differentiate postembolization infection or abscess from leukocytosis.[75]

Within the realm of neurologic embolization procedures, hemorrhage after embolization of meningiomas and arteriovenous malformations is a rare but potentially devastating complication. The causes of this phenomenon are unknown, but are thought to be due to abnormal vascular structure that gave rise to the malformation initially. Studies have shown that most of these bleeds are subarachnoid in nature.[77]

Many embolization procedures aim to eliminate blood flow to a portion of a diseased organ. Careful preprocedure evaluation is performed to ensure that there is enough functional tissue to maintain organ function after embolization. Nevertheless, acute failure of the organ is a possible complication. Monitoring laboratory indicators of function in the immediate postprocedure phase and for up to 4 weeks after is essential. Laboratory values should be correlated with clinical findings.[26,27]

Infection can develop at the catheter insertion site, and also at the target embolization site if an abscess forms in the location of necrosed tissue. Symptoms of infection include fever greater than 101°F (38.5°C) and pain out of proportion to treatment that is not relieved by standard analgesia.[71,73] Diagnosis is made with CT or ultrasound. Treatment usually involves antibiotics and, occasionally, drainage of the abscess or surgery.

Current research is focusing on decreasing nontarget embolization and reducing symptoms of PES. As new technologies and techniques are developed, the number of applications increases. New procedures are designed almost daily to fully use the minimally invasive nature of catheter-directed embolization. Surgeons, medical physicians, and radiologists collaborate to treat disorders previously thought inoperable, improving outcomes for all.

## SUMMARY

Embolization has multiple uses, from stopping excessive or unwanted blood flow to necrosing hypervascular tumors or other lesions, palliation of pain, or causing organ hypertrophy in preparation for surgery. Advances in technology have led to particles and coils that can compress to travel through microcatheters and then expand to occlude the lumen of the vessel once released. Greater control of coils and particles also reduces the side effects of nontarget embolization and tissue necrosis. Advances in glue and the use of temporary agents such as Gelfoam have also increased the number of applications available. Procedures can be performed in a planned, controlled environment, in conjunction with surgery or emergently. Side effects include PES, infection, bleeding and/or hematoma, and abscess or necrosis of organ or tissue. Nursing management in the periprocedural period is essential. The nurse has an important role in preprocedure evaluation of laboratory values and overall patient condition as well as patient education regarding what to expect. During the procedure, the nurse provides sedation and continual monitoring, administering anti-inflammatory agents, antibiotics, pain relief, and anxiolysis as needed, while assessing patient response. Postprocedure assessment for pain or other complications are also essential. The nurse's role in recognizing potential problems, addressing them, and evaluating and intervening both during and after the procedure is an essential one in improving outcomes for all patients undergoing embolotherapy.

## REFERENCES

1. Patel A, Soulen M. Agents for small vessel/tissue embolization and transcatheter tissue ablation. In: Baum S, Pentecost M, editors. Abrams' angiography and interventional radiology. 2nd edition. Philadelphia: Lippincott Williams & Wilkins; 2006. p. 169–75.

2. Yoon W, Kim J, Kim Y, et al. Bronchial and nonbronchial systemic artery embolization for life-threatening hemoptysis: a comprehensive review. Radiographics 2002;22:1395–409.

3. Darcy M. Management of lower gastrointestinal bleeding. In: Mauro M, Murphy K, Thomson K, et al, editors, Image-guided interventions, vol. 1. Philadelphia: Saunders Elsevier; 2008. p. 665–74.

4. McPherson S. Management of upper gastrointestinal hemorrhage. In: Mauro M, Murphy K, Thomson K, et al, editors, Image-guided interventions, vol. 1. Philadelphia: Saunders Elsevier; 2008. p. 675–89.

5. Baum S. Arteriographic diagnosis and treatment of gastrointestinal bleeding. In: Baum S, Pentecost M, editors. Abrams' angiography and interventional radiology. 2nd edition. Philadelphia: Lippincott Williams & Wilkins; 2006. p. 487–515.

6. Brinson G, Noone P, Mauro M, et al. Bronchial artery embolization for the treatment of hemoptysis in patients with cystic fibrosis. Am J Respir Crit Care Med 1998;157:1951–8.

7. Demello A. Uterine artery embolization. AORN J 2001;73(4):788–814.

8. Wong Y, Wang L, Ng C, et al. Mortality after successful transcatheter arterial embolization in patients with unstable pelvic fractures: rate of blood transfusion as a predictive factor. J Trauma 2000;49(1):71–5.

9. Spies J. Uterine fibroid embolization. In: Baum S, Pentecost M, editors. Abrams' angiography and interventional radiology. 2nd edition. Philadelphia: Lippincott Williams & Wilkins; 2006. p. 801–19.

10. Artinyan A, Nelson R, Soriano P, et al. Treatment response to transcatheter arterial embolization and chemoembolization in primary and metastatic tumors of the liver. HPB (Oxford) 2008;10:396–404.

11. Loewe C, Schindl M, Cejna M, et al. Permanent transarterial embolization of neuroendocrine metastases of the liver using cyanoacrylate and lipiodol: assessment of mid- and long-term results. AJR Am J Roentgenol 2003;180:1379–84.

12. Murthy R, Xiong H, Nunez R, et al. Yttrium 90 resin microspheres for the treatment of unresectable colorectal hepatic metastases after failure of multiple chemotherapy regimens: preliminary results. J Vasc Interv Radiol 2005;16:937–45.

13. Nabil M, Gruber T, Yakoub D, et al. Repetitive transarterial chemoembolization (TACE) of liver metastases from renal cell carcinoma: local control and survival results. Eur Radiol 2008;18:1456–63.

14. Wong C, Qing F, Savin M, et al. Reduction of metastatic load to liver after intraarterial hepatic yttrium-90 radioembolization as evaluated by [18F] fluorodeoxyglucose positron emission tomographic imaging. J Vasc Interv Radiol 2005;16:1101–6.

15. Donnelly L, Adams D, Bisset G III. Vascular malformations and hemangiomas: a practical approach in a multidisciplinary clinic. AJR Am J Roentgenol 2000; 174:597–608.

16. Yakes W, Rossi P, Odink H. Arteriovenous malformation management. Cardiovasc Intervent Radiol 1996;19:65–71.

17. Yakes W. Extremity venous malformations: diagnosis and management. Semin Intervent Radiol 1994;11(4):332–9.

18. Shlansky-Goldberg R, Solomon J. Perspectives on varicoceles management. In: Baum S, Pentecost M, editors. Abrams' angiography and interventional radiology. 2nd edition. Philadelphia: Lippincott Williams & Wilkins; 2006. p. 776–800.

19. Abushaban L, Uthaman B, Endrys J. Transcatheter coil closure of pulmonary arteriovenous malformations in children. J Interv Cardiol 2004;17(1):23–6.

20. Abulkhir A, Limongelli P, Healy A, et al. Preoperative portal vein embolization for major liver resection: a meta-analysis. Ann Surg 2008;247(1):49–58.

21. Cynamon J, Lerer D, Veith F, et al. Hypogastric artery coil embolization prior to endoluminal repair of aneurysms and fistula: buttock claudication, a recognized but possibly preventable complication. J Vasc Interv Radiol 2000;11(5):573–7.

22. Covey M, Tuorto S, Brody L, et al. Safety and efficacy of preoperative portal vein embolization with polyvinyl alcohol in 58 patients with liver metastases. AJR Am J Roentgenol 2005;185:1620–6.
23. Chang C, Singal A, Ganeshan S. Use of splenic artery embolization to relieve tense ascites following liver transplantation in a patient with paroxysmal nocturnal hemoglobinuria. Liver Transpl 2007;13:1532–7.
24. Lin P, Terramani T, Bush R, et al. Concomitant intraoperative renal artery embolization and resection of complex renal carcinoma. J Vasc Surg 2003;38(3):446–50.
25. Madoff D, Denys A, Wallace M, et al. Splenic arterial interventions: anatomy, indications, technical considerations, and potential complications. Radiographics 2005;25:S191–211.
26. Idowu O, Soulen M. Chemoembolization for hepatocellular carcinoma. In: Mauro M, Murphy K, Thomson K, et al, editors, Image-guided interventions, vol. 1. Philadelphia: Saunders Elsevier; 2008. p. 767–85.
27. Sofocleous C, Nascimento R. Embolotherapy for the management of liver malignancies other than hepatocellular carcinoma. In: Mauro M, Murphy K, Thomson K, et al, editors, Image-guided interventions, vol. 1. Philadelphia: Saunders Elsevier; 2008. p. 786–98.
28. Brown K. Bland embolization for hepatic malignancies. In: Mauro M, Murphy K, Thomson K, et al, editors, Image-guided interventions, vol. 1. Philadelphia: Saunders Elsevier; 2008. p. 809–18.
29. Forauer A, Kent E, Cwikiel W, et al. Selective palliative transcatheter embolization of bony metastases from renal cell carcinoma. Acta Oncol 2007;46:1012–8.
30. Ward J, Velling T. Transcatheter therapeutic embolization of genitourinary pathology. Rev Urol 2000;2(4):236–45.
31. Salem R, Lewandowski R, Roberts C, et al. Use of yttrium-90 glass microspheres (TheraSphere) for the treatment of unresectable hepatocellular carcinoma in patients with portal vein thrombosis. J Vasc Interv Radiol 2004;15:335–45.
32. Lustberg H, Pollak. Mechanical embolization agents. In: Mauro M, Murphy K, Thomson K, et al, editors, Image-guided interventions, vol. 1. Philadelphia: Saunders Elsevier; 2008. p. 176–86.
33. Cope C, Burke D, Meranze S. Atlas of interventional radiology. New York: Grower Medical Publishing; 1990.
34. Ray C, Bauer J. Embolization agents. In: Mauro M, Murphy K, Thomson K, et al, editors, Image-guided interventions, vol. 1. Philadelphia: Saunders Elsevier; 2008. p. 131–9.
35. Castenada-Zunig W. Interventional radiology. 2nd edition. Philadelphia: Williams and Wilkins; 1992, reprinted 1997.
36. Kessel D, Robertson I. Interventional radiology a survival guide. 2nd edition. Philadelphia: Saunders Elsevier; 2007.
37. Banovac F. Obstetric hemorrhage. In: Baum S, Pentecost M, editors. Abrams' angiography and interventional radiology. 2nd edition. Philadelphia: Lippincott Williams & Wilkins; 2006. p. 820–9.
38. Rossi P, Passariello R, Simonetti G. Control of a traumatic vertebral arteriovenous fistula by a modified Gianturco coil embolus system. Available at: http://www.ajronline.org/cgi/reprint/131/2/331.pdf. Accessed March 18, 2009.
39. Melissano G, Venturini M, Baccellieri D, et al. Distal embolization and proximal stent-graft deployment: a dual approach to endovascular treatment of ruptured superior gluteal artery aneurysm. Tex Heart Inst J 2008;35(1):50–3.
40. Varela M, Real M, Burrel M, et al. Chemoembolization of hepatocellular carcinoma with drug eluting beads: efficacy and doxorubicin pharmacokinetics. J Hepatol 2007;46:474–81.

41. Saad W, Waldman D. Management of postcatheterization pseudoaneurysms. In: Mauro M, Murphy K, Thomson K, et al, editors, Image-guided interventions, vol. 1. Philadelphia: Saunders Elsevier; 2008. p. 525–36.

42. Kandarpa K, Aruny J. Handbook of interventional radiologic procedures. 3rd edition. Philadelphia: Lippincott Williams & Wilkins; 2002.

43. Ryu C, Whang S, Suh D, et al. Percutaneous direct puncture glue embolization of high-flow craniofacial arteriovenous lesions: a new circular ring compression device with a beveled edge. AJNR Am J Neuroradiol 2007;28:528–30.

44. Hyung J, Kim S, Han J, et al. Transcatheter arterial embolization of unresectable renal cell carcinoma with a mixture of ethanol and iodized oil. Cardiovasc Intervent Radiol 1994;17:323–7.

45. Sadick N. Advances in the treatment of varicose veins: ambulatory phlebectomy, foam sclerotherapy, endovascular laser, and radiofrequency closure. Dermatol Clin 2003;25:443–55.

46. Rosen R, Blei F. Hemangiomas and vascular malformations. In: Baum S, Pentecost M, editors. Abrams' angiography and interventional radiology. 2nd edition. Philadelphia: Lippincott Williams & Wilkins; 2006. p. 1180–212.

47. Smith P. A personal method for foam sclerotherapy: technique and results. In: Bergan J, Cheng V, editors. Foam sclerotherapy a textbook. London: Royal Society of Medicine Press Ltd; 2008. p. 69–78.

48. Wollman J. The history of sclerosant foams: persons, techniques, patents and medical improvements. In: Bergan J, Cheng V, editors. Foam sclerotherapy a textbook. London: Royal Society of Medicine Press Ltd; 2008. p. 3–13.

49. Rosen R, Blei F. Interventional management of hemangiomas, arteriovenous fistula. In: Mauro M, Murphy K, Thomson K, et al, editors, Image-guided Interventions, vol. 1. Philadelphia: Saunders Elsevier; 2008. p. 585–604.

50. Fanelli F, Salvatori F, Rabuffi P, et al. Onyx, a liquid embolic material for the treatment of type II endoleaks and arterio-venous fistulas and malformations. Available at: http://www.aimsymposium.org/pdf/aim/2046.pdf. Accessed April 24, 2009.

51. Castenada F, Goodwin S, Swischuk JL, et al. Treatment of pelvic arteriovenous malformations with ethylene vinyl alcohol copolymer (Onyx). J Vasc Interv Radiol 2002;13:513–6.

52. Koconis K, Singh H, Soares G. Partial splenic embolization in the treatment of patients with portal hypertension: a review of the English language literature. J Vasc Interv Radiol 2007;18(4):463–81.

53. Boyer TD, Haskal ZJ. The role of transjugular intrahepatic portosystemic shunt in the management of portal hypertension. Hepatology 2005;41(2):386–400.

54. Choi Y, Yoon C, Park J, et al. Balloon-occluded retrograde transvenous obliteration for gastric variceal bleeding: its feasibility compared with transjugular intrahepatic portosystemic shunt. Korean J Radiol 2003;4(2):109–15.

55. Kiyosue H, Mori H, Matsumoto S, et al. Transcatheter obliteration of gastric varices. Radiographics 2003;23(4):911–20.

56. Sim J, Alejos J, Moore J. Techniques and applications of transcatheter embolization procedures in pediatric cardiology. J Interv Cardiol 2003;16(5):425–48.

57. Smith T. Endovascular therapy of cerebral arteriovenous malformations. In: Baum S, Pentecost M, editors. Abrams' angiography and interventional radiology. 2nd edition. Philadelphia: Lippincott Williams & Wilkins; 2006. p. 863–75.

58. Alexander M. Intracranial aneurysm therapy. In: Baum S, Pentecost M, editors. Abrams' angiography and interventional radiology. 2nd edition. Philadelphia: Lippincott Williams & Wilkins; 2006. p. 876–82.

59. Barnett B, Hughes A, Lin S, et al. In vitro assessment of EmboGel and UltraGel radiopaque hydrogels for the endovascular treatment of aneurysms. J Vasc Interv Radiol 2009;20:507–12.
60. D'Othee B, Rousseau H, Soula P, et al. Aortic stent grafting and side-branch embolization in an expanding chronic type B dissection. J Thorac Cardiovasc Surg 1999;118:1021–5.
61. Sheehan M, Hagino R, Canby E, et al. Type 2 endoleaks after abdominal aortic aneurysm stent grafting with systematic mesenteric and lumbar coil embolization. Ann Vasc Surg 2006;20(4):458–63.
62. Stone J, Evans AJ. In vitro assessment of aortic stent-graft integrity following exposure to onyx liquid embolic agent. J Vasc Interv Radiol 2009;20:107–12.
63. Venbrux A. Pelvic venous incompetence: pelvic congestion syndrome. In: Baum S, Pentecost M, editors. Abrams' angiography and interventional radiology. 2nd edition. Philadelphia: Lippincott Williams & Wilkins; 2006. p. 830–6.
64. Gupta S, Johnson M, Murthy R, et al. Hepatic arterial embolization and chemoembolization for the treatment of patients with metastatic neuroendocrine tumors: variables affecting response rates and survival. Cancer 2005;104(8): 1590–602.
65. Aliberti C, Benea G, Massimo T, et al. Chemoembolization (TACE) of unresectable intrahepatic cholangiocarcinoma with slow-release doxorubicin-eluting beads: preliminary results. Cardiovasc Intervent Radiol 2008. Available at: http://www. biocompatibles.com. Accessed May 26, 2009.
66. Rimon U, Duvdevani M, Garniek A, et al. Ethanol and polyvinyl alcohol mixture for transcatheter embolization of renal angiomyolipoma. AJR Am J Roentgenol 2006; 187:762–8.
67. Barth K. Preintervention assessment, intraprocedure management, postintervention care. In: Baum S, Pentecost M, editors. Abrams' angiography and interventional radiology. 2nd edition. Philadelphia: Lippincott Williams & Wilkins; 2006. p. 1–18.
68. Sasso C. Core curriculum for radiologic and imaging nursing. 2nd edition. Pensacola (FL): American Radiological Nurses Association; 2008.
69. Merten J, Burges W, Gray L. Prevention of contrast-induced nephropathy with sodium bicarbonate: a randomized controlled trial. JAMA 2004;291(19): 2328–34.
70. Marenzi G, Assanelli E, Marana I, et al. N-Acetylcysteine and contrast-induced nephropathy in primary angioplasty. N Engl J Med 2006;354(26):2773–82.
71. Hemingway A, Allison D. Complications of embolization; analysis of 410 procedures. Radiology 1988;166:669–72.
72. Paraskevas K, Koutsias S, Mikhailidis D, et al. Cholesterol crystal embolization: a possible complication of peripheral endovascular interventions. J Endovasc Ther 2008;15(5):614–25.
73. Leung D, Goin J, Sickles C, et al. Determinants of postembolization syndrome after hepatic chemoembolization. J Vasc Interv Radiol 2001; 12(3):321–6.
74. Toso C, Asthana S, Bigam A, et al. Reassessing selection criteria prior to liver transplantation for hepatocellular carcinoma utilizing the scientific registry of transplant recipients database. Hepatology 2009;49(3):832–8.
75. Ganguli S, Faintuch S, Salazar G, et al. Postembolization syndrome: changes in white blood cell counts immediately after uterine artery embolization. J Vasc Interv Radiol 2008;19:443–5.

76. Bendszus M, Monoranu C, Schutz A, et al. Neurologic complications after particle embolization of intracranial meningiomas. AJNR Am J Neuroradiol 2005;26: 1413–9.
77. Simon C, Yu R, Wong G, et al. Postembolization hemorrhage of a large and necrotic meningioma. AJNR Am J Neuroradiol 2004;25:506–8.

# Carbon Dioxide Digital Subtraction Angiography: An Alternative to Iodinated Contrast

James G. Caridi, MD, FSIR*, Irvin F. Hawkins, MD, FSIR

KEYWORDS

- Carbon dioxide • DSA • Contrast • Renal failure
- Contrast allergy • GI bleeding

## HISTORY

Using gas as an imaging agent is not a novel idea. It was used in the early 1900s when radiology was in its infancy. Air was injected into the peritoneum in an attempt to display the abdominal viscera and tumors on radiograph.[1] Because room air is comprised of gases that do not readily dissolve, some of the gas diffused into the venous system, resulting in toxic air emboli. It was then decided that $CO_2$, because of its more rapid solubility (20 times oxygen),[2–4] should be used for this purpose. $CO_2$ was originally used in 1914 for the visualization of the abdominal viscera and subsequently used in the evaluation of the retroperitoneum, inferior vena cava, and hepatic veins, as well as for the diagnosis of pericardial effusion.[2–5]

In the 1970s, a mishap with an angiographic injector led to the delivery of 30 mL of air into the celiac axis.[6] There were no untoward clinical consequences. However, it was noted that there was a negative image of the celiac axis and its branches on the films. As a result of these images, Hawkins[6] pioneered the intra-arterial use of $CO_2$. Initially the images were rudimentary. They were poor quality and obtaining them was labor intensive. However, with technological advancements such as digital subtraction angiography, stacking software, tilting tables and reliable delivery systems, $CO_2$ became viable as an angiographic imaging agent.[6]

There has been no financial support for this manuscript.
Shands Hospital, College of Medicine, University of Florida, Box 100374, Gainesville, FL 32610, USA
* Corresponding author.
E-mail address: caridj@radiology.ufl.edu

## UNIQUE PROPERTIES OF $CO_2$

The obvious difference between $CO_2$ and other contrast agents is that it is a gas and therefore it displays typical gaseous attributes. It is invisible, compressible, nonviscous, and buoyant. Because it is produced endogenously it is nontoxic, nonallergic, and lacks renal toxicity. Compared with $O_2$ it is 20 times more soluble and is rapidly dissolved in blood.

Like most gases, $CO_2$ is invisible, which is not a problem. The potential problem that arises, however, is contamination from other more occlusive invisible gases, most commonly room air. Consequently, to avoid embolic complications it is imperative that steps be taken to prevent contamination. This subject is discussed in the following sections.

Because $CO_2$ is compressible, hand delivery differs from liquid contrast. With liquid contrast, a forceful hand injection is best performed with a smaller syringe that generates more force. If delivering a gas with a low-volume syringe, however, the gas merely compresses and does not enter the catheter. For this reason it is essential to use a larger syringe. The gas still compresses but then delivers after compression if sufficient gas is present. For controlled delivery it is best to purge the catheter with a small volume of $CO_2$ before delivering the desired dose. As a result, there is no resistance and smooth facile delivery can be performed.

Unlike liquid iodinated contrast, $CO_2$ does not mix with blood. To render an accurate image, $CO_2$ must displace blood within the vessel, as it is a negative contrast that is enhanced with subtraction. $CO_2$ is buoyant. If all of the blood within the vessel is not displaced, $CO_2$ increases to the nondependent portion of the vessel (**Fig. 1**). The accuracy of the image obtained depends on the amount of blood displaced. For example, in larger vessels (aorta and iliac arteries), if an insufficient volume is injected, there is incomplete displacement of blood, resulting in diminished contrast and potentially a spurious image. Normal vessels may seem smaller and stenosis more significant than their true caliber. To circumvent this problem, either a larger amount of $CO_2$ must be administered, or the area of interest should be placed in the nondependent position to facilitate the positioning of gas in that vessel.

The viscosity of $CO_2$ is 1/400 that of iodinated contrast, which has diagnostic and interventional implications. $CO_2$ travels where the thicker more viscous contrast may not, thereby permitting visualization of abnormalities such as arteriovenous (AV) fistulas, collaterals, and arterial hemorrhage. Also easily visualized is the portal vein from intrahepatic parenchymal injection of $CO_2$. The low viscosity permits

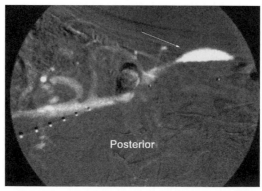

**Fig. 1.** Cross-table lateral flush $CO_2$ aortogram. Arrow indicates nondependent layering of $CO_2$ after injection. The patient's abdominal aortic aneurysm contributes to this positioning and may prelude accurate evaluation of the aorta.

passage of $CO_2$ into the hepatic sinusoids and subsequently into the portal vein. In addition, the low viscosity of $CO_2$ permits facile delivery through microcatheters, allowing easy visualization of small peripheral vessels.

As a result of its low viscosity, $CO_2$ delivery almost always results in reflux proximally or central to the catheter tip. Typically in iodinated contrast, when a selective injection is performed, the contrast travels peripheral to the catheter tip but rarely central. In many instances the central vascular structures and their pathologic condition are crucial to visualize and the use of $CO_2$ can be extremely advantageous. One of the best examples is with renal stent placement (**Fig. 2**). Once the selective catheter or balloon is placed beyond the renal artery stenosis a liquid contrast injection is effective only peripheral to the lesion. If $CO_2$ is delivered it will be effective more centrally and visualize the stenosis. $CO_2$ assists in more accurate stent positioning without the added potential complication of renal toxicity.

Advantages of $CO_2$ imaging

1. Nonallergic
2. Nonrenal toxic: can be given in unlimited quantities
3. Low viscosity
4. Reflux
5. Inexpensive: 1 mL = 0.005 cents.

Disadvantages of $CO_2$ imaging

1. It requires a unique delivery system
2. Bowel gas may obscure abdominal imaging
3. It is contraindicated in the cerebral arterial vessels
4. Accurate imaging can be more labor intensive.

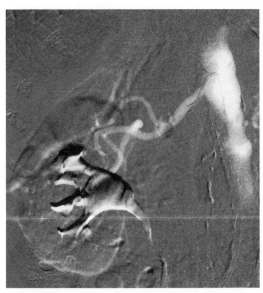

**Fig. 2.** Peripheral selective renal artery injection of $CO_2$ with reflux into the aorta. As opposed to iodinated contrast, this technique permits central visualization of the renal ostium, which facilitates accurate placement of renal stents.

## POTENTIAL COMPLICATIONS AND PRECAUTIONS
### Contamination

Because $CO_2$ is invisible, room air contamination can go undetected and result in occlusive gas emboli. In addition, our initial source of $CO_2$ was routine hospital stores. Our early injections had various clinical responses. When investigated, we found that old reusable $CO_2$ canisters were the source of water, rust, particulate matter, and carbonic acid. Typically, these are United States Pharmacopeia grade (99.5% pure) now used for laparoscopy. After this revelation, we changed to disposable Coleman or medical-grade $CO_2$ (99.99% pure), which resulted in nonpainful clinically reliable injections. Therefore, a pure medical-grade source and disposable cylinder are mandatory.

Furthermore, a closed delivery system is imperative to eliminate the additional possibility of room air contamination. Because of diffusivity and partial pressure differences of gases, an open system can result in $CO_2$ being replaced with less soluble room air over time. In addition, stopcocks should be at a minimum. Because of human error, they can be turned in the wrong direction, permitting the influx of room air. Even when turned appropriately, stopcocks are made for fluid not gas and gas may enter the system if a vacuum is created. Therefore, in our preferred system, we use 1-way valves to prevent human error and all valves and stopcocks are glued to eliminate the possibility of human error and room air aspiration.

### Excessive Volume

Excessive volume can be defined as one extremely large bolus of $CO_2$ or multiple smaller volumes given repetitively without sufficient time for $CO_2$ to resorb. Typically, we use a 35-mL syringe that is sufficient for imaging most vascular structures. Normally we wait 30 to 60 seconds between injections for $CO_2$ to absorb. Cho[7] showed that single injections of 1.6 mL/kg did not change pulmonary pressure, arterial pressure, $Po_2$, $Pco_2$, $Sao_2$, pH or lead to any clinical complications. Therefore 20 to 30 mL is well within the safety limits.

There are several caveats, however. Some systems connect the $CO_2$ canister directly to the delivery system. The $CO_2$ canisters contain approximately 3.3 million mL of $CO_2$ under high pressure. In these directly connected systems, the potential exists for inadvertent delivery of the contents of the canister because the pressure is higher than venous and arterial pressure. This error can have fatal consequences. Therefore, we advise never connecting the pressurized $CO_2$ canister directly to the delivery system. Also, it is important to allow sufficient time for resorption of the $CO_2$ before repeating injections. Typically 30 to 60 seconds is sufficient but this may be delayed in larger or aneurysmal vessels in which the blood gas interface is decreased. Fluoroscopy can generally be used to monitor for persistent gas.

In most instances increased volumes have no adverse affect but they do predispose for the possibility of trapping. If there is excessive volume of gas combined with a nondependent vessel or aneurysm, gas can become trapped and a vapor lock can ensue, preventing the flow of blood. Over time, the $CO_2$ is replaced with more occlusive nitrogen and oxygen, and ischemia can result. This is a rare phenomenon that can be avoided by taking the steps outlined earlier. In the rare occasion ischemia does occur, rolling the patient from side to side changes the dependency of the vessel involved and releases the gas. Others have suggested aspirating the gas with a catheter but we have not found this useful. We do check for trapped gas with fluoroscopy when we think a patient has susceptible anatomy.

### Explosive Delivery

Because $CO_2$ is compressible, there is a tendency to administer it as a rapid explosive injection. Typically the gas enters the syringe under pressure and compresses.

A 20-mL syringe can contain 200 mL of $CO_2$ if under pressure. The syringe is then connected to the delivery catheter either directly or by way of stopcocks or 1-way valves. If resistance is present in the catheter because of residual blood or saline, $CO_2$ compresses in the syringe before suddenly being forcefully delivered. In this scenario, we have shown that 95% of $CO_2$ is delivered in the last half second. We believe this type of delivery leads to rapid distension of the vessel and subsequent pain. The pain is more severe in veins where the muscular layer is not so well developed as arteries. In addition, explosive delivery of a compressed gas can lead to an unknown excessive volume being delivered, which can cause uncontrolled reflux and the potential for contamination of the central nervous system (CNS).[8]

Prevention of explosive delivery is simple. The delivery system should not be under pressure. The delivery syringe should aspirate a noncompressed volume of $CO_2$. Before its administration for diagnostic or therapeutic purposes, a small amount, approximately 5 mL, should be purged through the catheter. Following this procedure, there will be no resistance in the catheter and a known volume of $CO_2$ can be delivered in a controlled nonexplosive fashion.

## NITROUS OXIDE ANESTHESIA

$CO_2$ should be used with caution when using nitrous oxide anesthesia. In theory, nitrous oxide may diffuse from the soft tissue into the $CO_2$ gas bubble and cause a 5- to 6-fold increase in the occlusive effect.[9] Essentially, an innocuous 100-mL $CO_2$ bolus may have the effect of 500 to 600 mL of gas and result in a vapor lock.

### Chronic Obstructive Pulmonary Disease

Compared with the endogenous amount of $CO_2$ produced, approximately 250 mL/min, the amount delivered for diagnostic or therapeutic purposes is minimal. As long as the patient is not in respiratory failure, the small amounts of procedural vascular $CO_2$ should not have any detrimental effects.[10,11] As a safety precaution, however, we typically decrease the amount of bolus volume and wait longer between injections in those patients with tenuous chronic obstructive pulmonary disease.

### CNS Delivery

Arterial $CO_2$ delivery to the brain has had adverse effects in animals and humans.[8,12] It can cause breakdown of the blood-brain barrier and lead to ischemic infarction. We therefore avoid direct and indirect delivery to these vessels. Because of potential reflux and the possibility of flow to a nondependent position we never inject in the arterial system above the diaphragm. Venous delivery above the diaphragm is commonplace and not contraindicated.

Contraindications

1. Supradiaphragmatic arterial injections (intracranial $CO_2$)
2. Use with nitrous oxide anesthesia
3. Known right to left shunts.

Indications for $CO_2$ digital subtraction angiography (DSA)

1. Iodinated contrast allergies
2. Renal insufficiency
3. High-volume contrast procedures
4. Detection of arterial bleeding
5. Intervention.

$CO_2$ is nonallergic and therefore can be used whenever iodinated contrast is contra-indicated. This feature is especially useful in those emergency patients in whom a steroid preparation is not possible. It can also be useful in those scheduled allergic patients who have traveled a distance for a procedure and who may not have taken the preparation. Instead of disrupting or changing the schedule, $CO_2$ can be used as an alternative to iodinated contrast (**Fig. 3**).

Procedures previously considered contraindicated in patients with renal insufficiency can use all or mostly $CO_2$ as the contrast agent. We have used $CO_2$ in procedures that would otherwise risk putting the patient into renal failure, such as placing a transjugular intrahepatic portosystemic shunt (TIPS), uterine fibroid embolization, chemoembolization, and native and renal transplant artery evaluation. Any diagnostic or interventional arterial (excluding supradiaphragmatic procedures) or venous procedure can be performed using $CO_2$.

A common emergent procedure in which $CO_2$ is extremely valuable in either renal insufficiency or allergy is for inferior vena cava (IVC) filter placement. $CO_2$ is effective and comparable with iodinated contrast.[13,14] If an appropriate amount of $CO_2$ is delivered, it can accurately determine the size of the IVC. It is not so accurate for showing the renal veins or its variants. If, however $CO_2$ is deemed necessary and the imaging is substandard, renal vein location can be delineated by direct catheterization.[15]

$CO_2$ is especially valuable in renal artery intervention.[16] The closer iodinated contrast is injected to the renal artery the more renal toxic it becomes. Direct renal artery injection is the most damaging. $CO_2$ can replace iodinated contrast and be used with impunity, especially when multiple injections are necessary for precise stent placement. Similarly, $CO_2$ can be used without risk when evaluating and treating renal transplant arteries. $CO_2$ can supplement or supplant iodinated contrast in long high-volume procedures in patients with tenuous renal status.

Patients undergoing endovascular abdominal aneurysm repair (EVAR) have a propensity for developing renal failure,[17] including patients with and without preoperative renal dysfunction. It has been suggested that the incidence may even be greater than open repair. The population undergoing EVAR is usually more than 70 years old and these individuals have approximately a 30% incidence of abnormally low glomerular filtration rate, which may not be reflected by serum creatinine levels alone. Acute and delayed renal failure occurs after EVAR, with an acute incidence ranging from 7% to 25% when preexisting renal dysfunction is present and 2.5%

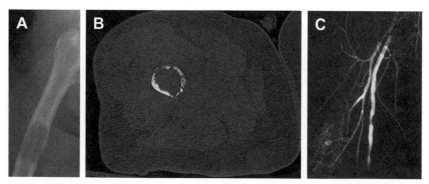

**Fig. 3.** (*A, B*) Plain film and computed tomography scan of a lytic renal cell metastatic lesion to the right femur requiring embolization before orthopedic repair. (*C*) $CO_2$ angiographic road map before embolization. The patient had renal compromise from previous removal of a renal cell carcinoma involving most of the right kidney.

when the creatinine is normal. Although not implicated as the only cause, iodinated contrast has been implicated as the major offender. Alternatively, $CO_2$ has been used as the major contrast agent by several investigators, allowing accurate and complete endovascular repair without inducing renal compromise.[18–20] In addition, it has also been suggested as a more sensitive agent for detecting endoleaks.

In the evaluation of acute arterial bleeding it has been shown that the use of $CO_2$ is twice as sensitive as its liquid counterpart. Hashimoto and colleagues[21,22] showed this increased sensitivity. There are basically 4 reasons for its increased visualization. As a gas, $CO_2$ is much less viscous than contrast and can escape more readily through a small rent in the artery. Also, $CO_2$ is usually under pressure in the artery and when it extravasates it expands in a cloudlike fashion, making it more visible (**Fig. 4**). As stated earlier it does not mix with blood so when it leaks out of the artery it does not dilute in the pool of extravasated blood. $CO_2$ does not have a capillary phase that can obscure small collections of gas.

When evaluating for gastrointestinal hemorrhage, bowel gas and patient motion can interfere and hamper interpretation.

As with arterial bleeding, $CO_2$ can also show AV fistulas more readily than iodinated contrast. The low viscosity permits more rapid and visible migration into the venous structures. It is highly sensitive for posttraumatic AV fistulas and often can be seen without selective cannulation of the feeding artery.[23,24] Considering the renal transplant postbiopsy AV fistula rate is 18%, $CO_2$ evaluation is effective in this scenario (**Fig. 5**).

Because of its low viscosity, when intraparenchymal injections of $CO_2$ are made into the liver, $CO_2$ travels into the sinusoids and opacifies the portal vein. This maneuver can assist in localizing the portal vein for portal vein embolization, thrombolysis,

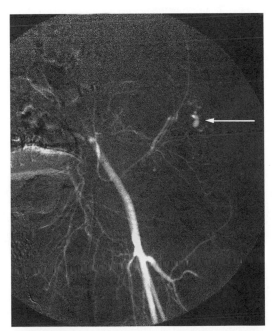

**Fig. 4.** Status of a 53-year-old patient after a motor vehicle accident with pelvic fractures now hemodynamically unstable. $CO_2$ nonselective angiogram (*arrow*) shows $CO_2$ extravasation, representing acute hemorrhage.

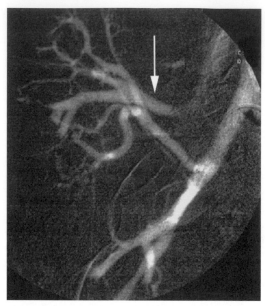

**Fig. 5.** Renal transplant patient status after biopsy with decreasing hematocrit and increasing creatinine. Arrow points to the venous limb of a posttraumatic renal AV fistula, shown by a nonselective $CO_2$ injection into the right common iliac vein.

TIPS, or any other portal intervention (**Fig. 6**). It avoids the potential fatal complications that have been reported in wedged $CO_2$ injections for portal vein visualization.[25] In a similar manner, $CO_2$ can be injected into the splenic pulp with a 25- or 27-guage spinal needle, resulting in imaging of the splenoportal system without a significant incidence of bleeding.

Likewise, a 25-guage needle can be placed in a peripheral extremity vein to perform extremity and chest venography. The low viscosity permits the use of a small-gauge needle and the lack of mixing with blood allows central visualization of the venous

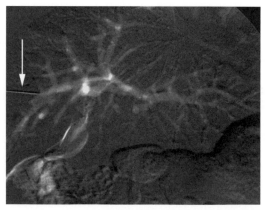

**Fig. 6.** Arrow points to a 22-guage needle in the liver parenchyma. 20 mL $CO_2$ was administered to visualize portal vein radicles and guide intervention.

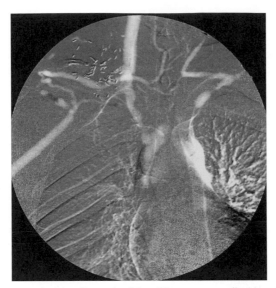

**Fig. 7.** A $CO_2$ venogram was performed with a 25-gauge needle in a right-hand vein to assess the central venous patency before central venous access placement. The attributes of $CO_2$ permit minimally invasive assessment of the presence of central veins and or their collateral pathways.

structures. We have used this for predialysis fistula evaluation as well as central venous angioplasty and stenting. $CO_2$ provides better imaging as it visualizes without dilution many of the smaller collateral veins (**Fig. 7**).

The viscosity of $CO_2$ allows facile injection into microcatheters, which results in better imaging of structures than forceful hand injection with liquid contrast. The small-caliber microcatheters combined with the viscous contrast often result in washed-out suboptimal images (**Fig. 8**).

The ability of $CO_2$ to reflux permits visualization central to the catheter tip that results in visualization of proximal stenosis when placing a stent or performing angioplasty. In addition, because of its low viscosity $CO_2$ can be injected through the catheter with a wire in place so that the guidewire does not have to be removed after an intervention. Follow-up angiography can be performed without losing access.

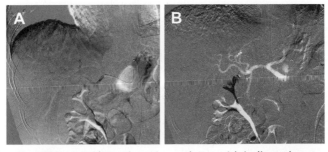

**Fig. 8.** (*A*) Hepatic arteriogram through a microcatheter with iodinated contrast as opposed to (*B*) with $CO_2$. The imaging in (*B*) is easier to perform and results in better visualization of the arteries.

## SUMMARY

$CO_2$ can be used in most vascular diagnostic or interventional procedures either by itself or as an adjunct to iodinated contrast. In some situations, delineated earlier, it may be more effective and useful even in the absence of allergy or renal insufficiency.

General delivery principles

Use a closed, nonpressurized system with limited stopcocks, glued connections, and 1-way valves.

Never leave a syringe filled with $CO_2$ open to room air as the $CO_2$ will be replaced by room air with time.

Never connect the delivery catheter directly to the $CO_2$ cylinder. This strategy avoids the potential inadvertent delivery of excessive and possibly lethal volumes of $CO_2$.

Avoid explosive delivery. Purging the delivery catheter of blood or saline results in a more controlled, smooth delivery with less discomfort and reflux.

Begin with small volumes injections of $CO_2$. Increase or decrease volume as required for specific anatomy.

Larger vessels require higher volumes of $CO_2$ to render a more accurate image; 30 to 35 mL is sufficient in most flush procedures. If a suboptimal image is rendered turn the desired area to the nondependent position.

Vessels equal to or less than 10 mm usually have a 1:1 correlation with contrast because 20 mL of $CO_2$ displaces most if not all of the blood in these sized vessels.

Wait 30 to 60 seconds between injections to allow any trapped $CO_2$ to dissolve.

Elevate the area of interest in poor flow conditions (feet, 10–15°; renal artery, 30–45°).

Vasodilators (nitroglycerin 100–150 μg intra-arterially) can be used to improve filling in the extremities.

End-hole catheters deliver most consistent bolus of $CO_2$.

DSA imaging principles

5 to 7 frames/s using a 60-ms pulse width with adequate penetration

To reduce the bubbling effect of $CO_2$, when necessary use a stacking program that superimposes multiple frames to yield a composite image

Glucagon can be used to reduce bowel gas motion.

$CO_2$ may not be the consummate imaging agent but with a little preparation and learning it can be extremely useful when used alone or in conjunction with iodinated contrast in those situations in which traditional contrast fails or is contraindicated.

## REFERENCES

1. Rautenberg E. Rontgenphotographie der Leber, der Milz, und des Zwerchfells. Dtsch Med Wochenschr 1914;24:1205 [in German].
2. Rosenstein P. Pneumoradiology of kidney position–a new technique for the radiological representation of the kidneys and neighboring organs (suprarenal gland, spleen, liver). J Urol 1921;15:447.
3. Paul RE, Durant TM, Oppenheiner MJ, et al. Intravenous carbon dioxide for intracardiac gas contrast in the roentgen diagnosis of pericardial effusion and thickening. Am J Roentgenol Radium Ther Nucl Med 1957;78:224–5.

4. Carelli HH, Sorddelli E. A new procedure for examining the kidney. Rev Asoc Med Argent 1921;34:18.
5. Phillips JH, Burch GE, Hellinger R. The use of intracardiac carbon dioxide in the diagnosis of pericardial disease. AJR Am J Roentgenol 1966;97:342–9.
6. Hawkins IF. Carbon dioxide digital subtraction angiography. AJR Am J Roentgenol 1982;139:19–24.
7. Cho KJ. Venous application of $CO_2$ (clinical and experimental). Presented at the Annual Meeting of Advances in Vascular Interventional and $CO_2$ Angiography. New York, May 30–31, 1997.
8. Ehrman KO, Taber TE, Gaylord GM, et al. Comparison of diagnostic accuracy with carbon dioxide versus iodinated contrast material in the imaging of hemodialysis access fistulas. J Vasc Interv Radiol 1980;52:52–5.
9. Steffey EP, Johnson BH, Eger EI. Nitrous oxide intensifies the pulmonary arterial pressure response to venous injection of carbon dioxide in the dog. Anesthesiology 1980;52:52–5.
10. Weaver FA, Pentecost MJ, Yellin AE. Carbon dioxide digital subtraction arteriography: a pilot study. Ann Vasc Surg 1990;4:437–41.
11. Frankhouse JG, Ryan MG, Papanicoaon G, et al. Carbon dioxide digital subtraction arteriography – assisted transluminal angioplasty. Ann Vasc Surg 1995;9(5):448–52.
12. Coffey R, Quisling R, Mickle JP, et al. The cerebrovascular effects of intraarterial $CO_2$ in quantities required for diagnostic imaging. Radiology 1984;151:405–10.
13. Sullivan KL, Bonn J, Shapiro MJ, et al. Venography with carbon dioxide as a contrast agent. Cardiovasc Intervent Radiol 1995;18:141–5.
14. Holtzman R, Lottenberg L, Bass T. Comparison of carbon dioxide and iodinated contrast for cavography prior to inferior vena cava filter placement. Am J Surg 2003;185:364–8.
15. Boyd-Kranls R, Sullivan K, Eschelman D, et al. Accuracy and safety of carbon dioxide inferior vena cavography. J Vasc Interv Radiol 1999;10:1183–9.
16. Caridi JG, Stavropolous W, Hawkins IF. $CO_2$ digital subtraction angiography for renal artery angioplasty in high-risk patients. AJR Am J Roentgenol 1999;173:1551–6.
17. Walsh SR, Tang TY, Boyle J. Renal consequences of endovascular abdominal aortic aneurysm repair. J Endovasc Ther 2008;15:73–82.
18. Chao A, Major K, Kumar SR, et al. Carbon dioxide digital subtraction angiography-assisted endovascular aortic aneurysm repair in the azotemic patient. J Vasc Surg 2007;45:451–60.
19. Gahlen J, Hansmann J, Hardy S, et al. Carbon dioxide angiography for endovascular grafting in high risk patients with infrarenal abdominal aortic aneurysms. J Vasc Surg 2001;33:646–9.
20. Criado E, Kabbani L, Cho K. Catheter-less angiography for endovascular aortic aneurysm repair: a new application of carbon dioxide as a contrast agent. J Vasc Surg 2008;48:527–34.
21. Hashimoto S, Hiramatsu K, Sato M. $CO_2$ as an intra-arterial digital subtraction angiography agent in the management of trauma. Semin Intervent Radiol 1997;14:163–73.
22. Hashimoto S. Detection of bleeding in $CO_2$ DSA. Presented at the Third Annual Meeting of the Congress of the Asia-Pacific Society of Cardiovascular and Interventional Radiology. Melbourne, Australia, April 6–11, 1997.
23. Moresco KP, Patel NH, Namyslowski Y. Carbon dioxide angiography of the transplanted kidney. Technical considerations and imaging findings. AJR Am J Roentgenol 1998;171:1271–6.

24. Takeda T, Ido K, Yuasa Y, et al. Intraarterial digital subtraction angiography with carbon dioxide: superior detectability of arteriovenous shunting. Cardiovasc Intervent Radiol 1988;11:101–7.
25. Semba DP, Saperstein L, Nyman U, et al. Hepatic laceration from wedged venography performed before transjugular intrahepatic portosystemic shunt placement. J Vasc Interv Radiol 1996;7:143–6.

# Evidence-Based Acute Management of Sepsis—Rapid Intervention in the Critical Hours

Jeffrey P. Gonzales, PharmD, BCPS[a],*, Lou-Ellen Lallier, MS, CRNP[b]

**KEYWORDS**

- Sepsis • Severe sepsis • Fluid resuscitation • Vasopressors
- Antibiotics

## CASE PRESENTATION

A 36-year-old Caucasian man with a history of diverticulitis presented to the emergency department with severe abdominal pain, fever (38.3°C), nausea, and abdominal rigidity. A stat computed tomographic scan revealed severe diverticulitis with intestinal rupture, and he underwent an emergent colon resection. Postoperatively, he was placed in the surgical intermediate care unit for monitoring. By postoperative day 2, the patient's abdominal pain worsened, he was febrile (39.5°C), tachycardic (120 beats per minute), tachypneic (22 breaths per minute), and hypotensive (blood pressure of 80/43 mm Hg; mean arterial blood pressure [MAP] of 55 mm Hg). His oxygen saturation via pulse oximeter decreased to 95% on room air, his urine output decreased to 10 mL/h, and the urine was hazy and dark amber. His skin was cool with a capillary refill time of 4 seconds. On further examination, his surgical site was erythematous and edematous with purulent drainage. The nurse immediately applied 2 L oxygen via nasal cannula and notified the surgical team. One liter of normal saline was administered, and the nurse in charge sent stat laboratory panels. The results were as follows: white blood cell (WBC) count, 23,000 cells/$\mu$L; hemoglobin, 10 g/dL; hematocrit, 29%; platelets, 125 × 10$^3$/$\mu$L; sodium, 145 mEq/L; potassium, 3.9 mEq/L; chloride, 102 mEq/L; bicarbonate, 36 mEq/L; *blood urea nitrogen*, 32 mg/dL; creatinine, 2.0 mg/dL; glucose, 152 mg/dL; and lactate, 6 mg/dL.

[a] Critical Care, Department of Pharmacy Practice and Science, University of Maryland School of Pharmacy, 20 North Pine Street, Room 443, Baltimore, MD 21201, USA
[b] Medical Intensive Care Unit, University of Maryland Medical Center, 22 South Green Street, Baltimore, MD 21201, USA
* Corresponding author.
*E-mail address:* jgonzale@rx.umaryland.edu

Perioperative Nursing Clinics 5 (2010) 189–202
doi:10.1016/j.cpen.2010.02.003                    **periopnursing.theclinics.com**
1556-7931/10/$ – see front matter © 2010 Elsevier Inc. All rights reserved.

The incidence, morbidity, and mortality of sepsis and severe sepsis are increasing in the United States.[1,2] The reasons for the increased incidence of sepsis are unknown, but it may be related to an aging population, more intravenous catheters in the community, and/or more immunocompromised patients.[2,3] A large 22-year study on the epidemiology of sepsis in the United States reported a dramatic increase in sepsis from 82.7 cases per 100,000 population in 1979 to more than 240 cases per 100,000 population in 2000.[1] Even with today's best practices, the mortality rate of sepsis is unacceptably high, ranging from 30% to 40%.[1–3] Recent data suggest that more than 500 people die of sepsis daily in the United States.[1] Most patients who die from sepsis would have developed some form of multiorgan failure. The most common severe organ failures associated with sepsis are acute respiratory distress syndrome, shock, acute renal failure, and neurologic failure (mental status change, coma).[4] The cost associated with sepsis is enormous, most of which is generated from the intensive-care-unit (ICU) stay, the emergency department, and the operating rooms. The average length of stay for patients with sepsis approaches 20 days, with a cost of more than $22,000. The national hospital cost associated with the care of severe sepsis in the United States is more than $16 billion.[1]

The Institute of Health Care in conjunction with the Surviving Sepsis Campaign has put forth considerable efforts to improve sepsis treatment, with the goal of reducing mortality. The Surviving Sepsis Campaign published their most recent evidence-based guidelines in 2008.[5] These guidelines support the early detection of sepsis, prompt and aggressive resuscitation, broad-spectrum antibiotic therapy, and source control. The guidelines have 2 levels of recommendations; Grade 1 indicates a strong recommendation, whereas Grade 2 indicates a weak recommendation. The guidelines also use letters denoting the level of evidence: A, high; B, moderate; C, low; D, very low. For example, Grade 1C is a strong recommendation with low-level evidence.[5] Others have shown that the implementation of these evidence-based guidelines and protocols has led to a reduction in mortality and morbidity.[6,7]

This review provides an evidence-based approach for the acute management of sepsis and severe sepsis, focusing primarily on the initial critical hours. The review covers evaluation and diagnosis, fluid resuscitation, antibiotic therapy, source control, and vasopressors/inotropic agents. Adjunctive therapies (steroid replacement, activated protein C, tight glycemic control, nutrition, deep venous thromboprophylaxis, and stress ulcer prophylaxis) are out of the scope of this review. However, these adjunctive therapies should be considered within the first 24 to 48 hours of presentation for optimal management.

## EVALUATION AND DIAGNOSIS

Sepsis is classically defined as an infection in addition to at least 2 of the systemic inflammatory response syndrome (SIRS) findings (**Box 1**). Severe sepsis is sepsis associated with any acute organ failure (neurologic, pulmonary, cardiovascular, renal, hepatic, and/or metabolic), hypoperfusion (lactate>2 mg/dL, decreased capillary refill time, mottled skin), or hypotension (MAP<70 mm Hg or requiring vasopressors). Septic shock is sepsis with hypotension that is refractory to adequate fluid resuscitation (at least 15 mL/kg of crystalloid fluid).[8] In fact, the disease is a continuum, from an infection to the development of sepsis in some patients to the development of organ failure (severe sepsis) and/or possible shock, and finally resolution or death. Other common clinical signs of sepsis/infection are acute mental status changes, decreased urine output, hypotension, decreased skin perfusion, and hyperglycemia (serum glucose>140 mg/dL).[8] The most common sources of infection in sepsis are respiratory

---

**Box 1**
**Clinical signs of sepsis**

SIRS

- Fever (>38.3°C) or hypothermia (<36°C)
- Tachycardia (>90 beats/min)
- Tachypnea (>20 breaths/min or hyperventilation [$Paco_2$<32])
- White blood cell count of more than 12,000 cells/μL or less than 4000 cells/μL or presence of more than 10% neutrophils

Other clinical features of sepsis

- Acute organ failure

  Neurologic

  1. Altered mental status

  Pulmonary

  1. Increased respiratory rate

  2. Decreased oxygen saturation

  3. $Pao_2/Fio_2$ less than 300

  Cardiovascular

  1. Systolic blood pressure less than 90 mm Hg

  2. MAP less than 70 mm Hg

  Renal

  1. Urine output less than 0.5 mL/kg/h

  2. Creatinine increase more than 0.5 mg/dL

  Hepatic

  1. Impaired coagulation (international normalized ratio>1.5 or a *partial thromboplastin time*>60 seconds)

  2. Thrombocytopenia (platelet <100,000/μL)

  3. Hyperbilirubinemia (serum bilirubin>4 mg/dL)

  Metabolic

  1. Lactate more than 2 mmol/L

  2. Hyperglycemia (serum glucose>140 mg/dL)

- Hypoperfusion
- Decreased capillary refill time

---

infections (61%), blood stream infections (18.5%), abdominal infections (8.6%), and genitourinary infections (6.8%).[4]

Nurses who suspect sepsis in their patients, based on clinical findings (eg, fever, tachycardia, hypotension, increased WBC count, change in mental status, decreased perfusion), should obtain at least 2 blood cultures before initiating antibiotics to optimize obtaining microbiology data (Grade IC).[5] However, obtaining blood cultures should not delay prompt antibiotic treatment for suspected sepsis. At least 1 blood culture should be drawn peripherally, and in patients with central catheters, at least

1 blood culture should be drawn through the device. In addition to culturing blood, other possible sites of infection should be cultured as necessary (eg, urine, cerebral spinal fluid, abscesses, and secretions). Imaging studies should be performed to help confirm diagnosis when clinically safe (Grade 1C). Imaging studies may also help to determine if the patient is a surgical candidate (drainage of abscess, removal of foreign body, debridement of wounds, or other procedures).[5] There are some data suggesting the use of biomarkers (ie, procalcitonin and C-reactive protein) to help with the early identification of sepsis.[9,10] However, these methods are still in the investigational phase and cannot be routinely recommended.[11,12]

## FLUID RESUSCITATION

After stabilization of the patient (ABCs: airway, breathing, circulation), the initial goal is to assess and restore tissue perfusion with early aggressive resuscitation (Grade 1C).[5] Fluid resuscitation alone may improve cardiac output and hypotension in patients who are volume depleted. Patients with subclinical hypoperfusion (not hypotensive and with normal mental status) may seem stable; however, these patients still need early aggressive resuscitation.[13] Early resuscitation has been shown to decrease mortality and morbidity in severe sepsis. The landmark Early Goal-Directed Therapy (EGDT) study showed that aggressive early resuscitation using goal-directed therapy dramatically decreases mortality and morbidity.[14] Since the publication of that study, others have duplicated their findings in different clinical settings.[6,15] The implementation of EGDT improves outcomes in septic shock and should be considered as soon as sepsis is identified (Grade 1C).[5] EGDT uses endpoints to optimize fluid resuscitation, including central venous pressure (CVP; goal, 8–12 mm Hg), MAP (goal $\geq$ 65 mm Hg), urine output (goal $\geq$ 0.5 mL/kg/h), and mixed venous or central venous saturation (goal $\geq$ 65% or 70%, respectively) (**Fig. 1**). Other indices of perfusion may be used, such as change in mental status, cool skin and decreased capillary refill, and elevated serum lactate concentrations.[5,16]

There are many techniques to assess intravascular volume in the critically ill, such as measurement of CVP, pulmonary artery occlusion pressure (PAOP) obtained from a pulmonary artery catheter, left ventricular end-diastolic area via echocardiography, and stroke volume variation. Each of these measures has its own limitations, but they can be useful to the clinician to guide fluid therapy in the critically ill population. Frequent reassessment of these endpoints should be performed in case of ongoing hypoperfusion and/or septic shock.[5,16–18]

The choice of fluid for resuscitation remains controversial; however, initial resuscitation is usually performed by infusing large volumes of crystalloid fluids (normal saline or lactated Ringer solution) followed by colloids (albumin or starches). The Surviving Sepsis Guidelines recommend either crystalloids or colloids for the initial resuscitation fluid (Grade 1B).[5] With either fluid, it is recommended to resuscitate to an initial target CVP of 8 mm Hg or more (or 12 mm Hg in patients under mechanical ventilation) (Grade 1C). Fluid resuscitation should be separated from general maintenance fluid needs of the patient. Fluid boluses or challenges are preferred to continuous fluid administration (Grade 1D). Using the fluid challenge method, clinicians can get a better evaluation of hemodynamic responsiveness and cardiac filling pressures compared with continuous fluid administration. Fluid challenges should be administered rapidly in volumes of approximately 500 to 1000 mL for crystalloids and 300 to 500 mL for colloids. Volume status, blood pressure, perfusion, and oxygenation should be evaluated after every bolus. In patients with limited ventricular function, these volumes may be reduced. Fluid administration should continue during hypoperfusion and shock and

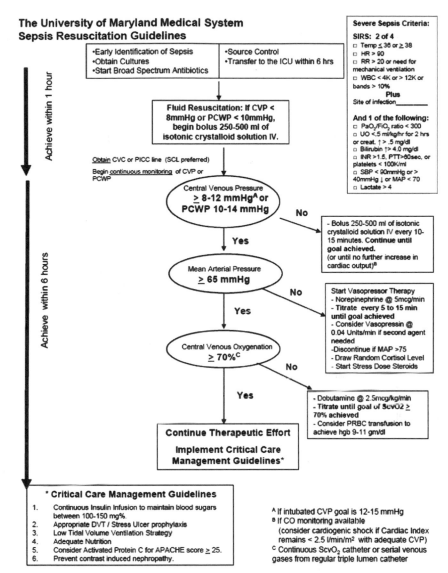

**Fig. 1.** Resuscitation. CVC, central venous catheter; DVT, deep vein thrombosis; HR, heart rate; INR, international normalized ratio; PCWP, pulmonary capillary wedge pressure; PICC, peripherally inserted central catheter; PRBC, packed red blood cells; RR, respiratory rate; SBP, systolic blood pressure; SCL, subclavian line. (*Courtesy of* Avelino C. Verceles, MD, Assistant Professor of Medicine, University of Maryland, Pulmonary and Critical Care Medicine.)

should be reduced only when (1) there is evidence of increased cardiac filling pressures (CVP or PAOP) without improvement in systemic blood pressure, (2) there is normalization of clinical end points of blood pressure (heart rate, MAP, increased urine output), or (3) there is evidence of pulmonary congestion.[5] Large volumes (>6–10 L of crystalloid fluid) may be needed in the first 24 hours of septic shock.[16] In fact, in the EGDT study, an average of 5 L of fluid was administered in the first 6 hours of presentation compared with an average of 3.5 L of fluid in the standard therapy.[14]

The Saline versus Albumin Fluid Evaluation (SAFE) study investigators evaluated the administration of crystalloids (normal saline) versus 4% albumin in a large (approximately 7000 patients) randomized, multicenter study in the critically ill population. The study concluded that 4% albumin was equally effective (no difference in mortality or new organ failure) and as safe as crystalloids. There was a trend in benefit for normal saline in the trauma population and a trend in benefit for albumin in the population with acute respiratory disease. However, further studies evaluating the use of albumin in these specific populations are needed before its use can be routinely recommended.[19]

Classically, it has been taught that 4 times as much crystalloid is needed to produce the same effect as colloids. However, in the SAFE study, the albumin to crystalloid ratio (1:1.4) was lower than in previous studies.[19] Isotonic crystalloid solutions (0.9% normal saline) generally expand the intravascular space by roughly 20% to 25% of volume infused. For example, for every liter of crystalloid solution infused, 200 to 250 mL remains in the intravascular space (**Table 1**).[20] Five percent albumin or a similar concentration of colloid/starch increases the intravascular space by as much as the amount infused. For example, 500 mL of 5% albumin increases the intravascular space by approximately 500 mL. Because of the increase in oncotic pressures of higher concentration albumin, 25% albumin increases the intravascular space 3 to 5 times the amount infused.[20] However, patients with sepsis generally have a significant amount of increased vascular permeability. Therefore, the amount of fluid mobilized from the interstitial space to the intravascular space may be minimized.[21] However, in severe increases of vascular permeability, an increased amount of fluid can also be mobilized from the intravascular space into the interstitial space, reducing the effectiveness of crystalloid and/or colloid resuscitation and causing third spacing of the fluid.[21]

After fluid resuscitation is complete and there is resolution of hemodynamic compromise and improved perfusion, there are data to suggest a more conservative fluid-management strategy. The Acute Respiratory Distress Syndrome Network studied 2 fluid-management strategies in acute lung injury, conservative and liberal fluid management. To achieve a conservative fluid balance, the study actively diuresed the patients, while using endpoints such as CVP, urine output, and overall fluid balance. This method has been shown to significantly decrease time on the mechanical ventilator and ICU length of stay, without additional risk to the patient, and should be considered in patients who are hemodynamically stable.[22]

## ANTIBIOTIC THERAPY

Prompt broad-spectrum empiric antibiotics are recommended in patients presenting with presumed or documented sepsis (Grade 1B).[5] There are data that suggest that

**Table 1**
**Response and duration of volume expansion**

| Solution | Volume Expansion[a] (%) | Duration of Expansion (h) | Plasma Half-Life (h) |
|---|---|---|---|
| 0.9% Sodium Chloride | 20–25 | 1–4 | 0.5 |
| Lactated Ringer | 20–25 | 1–4 | 0.5 |
| 5% Albumin | 70–100 | 12–24 | 16–24 |
| 25% Albumin | 300–500 | 12–24 | 16–24 |

[a] Percentage of administered volume.

*Data from* American Thoracic Society. Evidence-based colloid use in the critically ill: American Thoracic Society Consensus Statement. Am J Respir Crit Care Med 2004;170:1247–59.

early administration of antibiotics improves patient outcomes, especially when administered in the first hour of presentation in septic shock (Grade 1B) and severe sepsis (Grade 1D).[5,23,24] Delays in appropriate antibiotic therapy have been shown to increase mortality and morbidity.[23,25] In general, the clinician should have knowledge of the suspected source of sepsis, have understanding of what the common microbes or yeast/fungi for the different sources are (**Table 2**), and have an understanding of the spectrum of coverage of the antibiotic chosen. Institution-specific susceptibilities and antibacteriograms are extremely important when choosing empiric antibiotics. When microbiology susceptibility data are available, it is recommended to de-escalate the antibiotic therapy to the narrowest spectrum antibiotics that are effective against the organism. The guidelines suggest a daily reassessment of antibiotics to optimize efficacy; to decrease resistance, adverse effects, and costs; and to narrow therapy (Grade 1C). There are inadequate data to routinely recommend double coverage of antibiotics; however, Surviving Sepsis Campaign suggests considering double coverage in patients with known or suspected pseudomonal infections (Grade 2D).[5]

Ideally, antibiotics should be initiated after cultures are drawn. For the critically ill patient, a common regimen includes (1) carbapenem (imipenem, meropenem, or doripenem), a third or fourth generation cephalosporin (ceftriaxone or cefepime), or an extended spectrum β-lactam antibiotic (piperacillin-tazobactam) with or without an aminoglycoside, (2) atypical coverage (a macrolide or floroquinolone), and (3) an agent that covers gram-positive organisms that may be resistant to β-lactams (ie, methicillin-resistant *Staphylococcus aureus* [MRSA], vancomycin-resistant enterococci [VRE]). It is important to evaluate the patient for the potential for resistant organisms, as this affects the antibiotics chosen.

There are few studies that specifically evaluate the duration of antibiotic therapy in the critically ill.[26] As a general rule, as long as there is improvement in the patient's condition (eg, absence of fever, decreased WBC count, hemodynamic stability), 7 to 10 days of antibiotics is sufficient for most cases (Grade 1D).[5] Longer duration of therapies may be applicable to deep-seeded infections or for infections that are difficult to eradicate based on the source (abscesses, osteomyolitis, endocarditis, MRSA pneumonia, or infections with nonfermenting gram-negative organisms).[26–28]

| Table 2 | |
| --- | --- |
| **Common organisms for potential sources** | |
| **Source** | **Common Organisms** |
| Lung | |
| Community | *Streptococcus pneumonia, Haemophilus influenza, Moraxella catarrhalis, Mycoplasma* spp, *Chlamydia pneumonia, Legionella* |
| Nosocomial | *Pseudomonas aeruginosa, Acinetobacter baumannii, Enterobacter* spp, *Serratia* spp, *Proteus* spp, *Klebsiella* spp, *Staphylococcus aureus* |
| Urine | *Escherichia coli, Proteus mirabilis, Staphylococcus* spp, other gram-negative organisms, and yeasts/fungi |
| Catheter | *Staphylococcus* spp, *Streptococcus* spp, *Enterococcus* spp, gram-negative organisms, and yeasts/fungi |
| Central Nervous System | *Streptococcus pneumonia, Haemophilus influenza, Neiserria meningicoccus, Listeria* spp, *Staphylococcus* spp (if catheter), gram-negative organisms (if catheter) |

## SOURCE CONTROL

The overall goal for source control is the rapid diagnosis of sepsis and the identification of possible sites of infection to eliminate the source when possible. Source control is a vital component of early sepsis care and can be as important as antibiotic therapy, especially in diseases such as necrotizing fasciitis, intraabdominal abscesses, ischemic bowel, toxic megacolon, or severe *Clostridium difficile* colitis, perforated viscus, ascending cholangitis, infectious necrotizing pancreatitis, infectious empyema, foreign body infections, and obstructive uropathy or complicated pyelonephritis. In these cases, prompt surgical intervention may be needed, and the timeliness of intervention is associated with better outcomes. Source control can also be accomplished by the removal of any suspected infected intravascular or tunneled device. In general, fluid resuscitation should begin before the identification of the infectious source (Grade 1C). The Surviving Sepsis Guidelines recommend that all patients be evaluated for infections that could benefit from source control (eg, abscess drainage, wound debridement, infected device removal; Grade 1C). The site of infection should be established as early as possible (Grade 1C) and within 6 hours of presentation (Grade 1D). When source control is necessary, the intervention with the least amount of potential insult should be used (Grade 1D). Intravascular devices that are potential sources should be removed after additional intravenous access has been obtained (Grade 1C).[5]

## VASOPRESSORS/INOTROPIC AGENTS

After fluid resuscitation is initiated and fails to reestablish normal blood pressure ($\geq$65 mm Hg, Grade 1C) and tissue perfusion, vasopressors should be administered to help maintain perfusion.[5] Vasopressor agents fall into 2 categories, catecholamine vasopressors and vasopressin agonists. Catecholamine vasopressors are the most routinely used in clinical practice. The catecholamine vasopressors (norepinephrine, dopamine, phenylephrine, and epinephrine) have strong vasoconstrictive properties with varying activities on the beta and alpha receptors (**Table 3**). The main vasoconstrictive properties of catecholamine vasopressors are the result of alpha stimulation on blood vessels (increased systemic vascular resistance and blood pressure). In addition to the stimulation of alpha receptors, some of the catecholamine vasopressors also bind to the beta-1 receptors, causing an increase in force of cardiac contractility (increased cardiac output) and rate of cardiac contractility (increased heart rate). Furthermore, some catecholamine vasopressors (dobutamine) bind to the beta-2 receptors, causing dilation of the vasculature (may cause hypotension) (see **Table 3**). The only clinically used vasopressin agonist available in the United States is vasopressin. All of the catecholamine vasopressors can be rapidly titrated (every 5–10 minutes) to achieve goal MAP. Norepinephrine and dopamine should be considered first-line vasopressors (Grade 1C), followed by vasopressin (Grade 2C). In refractory septic shock states, phenylephrine and/or epinephrine should be administered (Grade 2C).[5]

Norepinephrine is primarily an alpha agonist, with high receptor affinity for the alpha receptor. Although norepinephrine has minimal beta receptor effects, tachycardia may result with norepinephrine use, especially at higher doses and with intravascular volume depletion. Norepinephrine should be started at a low dose (0.01–0.05 μg/kg/min) and titrated every 5 to 10 minutes to maintain normal blood pressures. Norepinephrine is considered to have stronger vasoconstrictor effects when compared with dopamine and has a wide dosing range (0.01–3.3 μg/kg/min). There are some studies to suggest that norepinephrine maintains gastric and renal perfusion after fluid

**Table 3**
**Vasopressor receptor activity**

| Vasopressor Agent | Receptor Binding | | | | | |
|---|---|---|---|---|---|---|
| | $\alpha_1$ | $\alpha_2$ | $\beta_1$ | $\beta_2$ | $DA_1$ | $V_1$ |
| Dopamine (μg/kg/min) | | | | | | |
| 1–3 | 0 | 0 | + | 0 | ++++ | 0 |
| 3–10 | 0/+ | 0 | ++++ | ++ | ++++ | 0 |
| 10–25 | +++ | 0 | ++++ | + | 0 | 0 |
| Norepinephrine (μg/kg/min) | | | | | | |
| 0.01–3.3 | +++ | ++ | + | + | 0 | 0 |
| Phenylephrine (μg/kg/min) | | | | | | |
| 0.25–8 | +++ | + | ? | 0 | 0 | 0 |
| Epinephrine (μg/kg/min) | | | | | | |
| 0.01–0.05 | ++ | ++ | ++++ | +++ | 0 | 0 |
| >0.05–2 | ++++ | ++++ | +++ | + | 0 | 0 |
| Vasopressin | | | | | | |
| 0.04 U/min | 0 | 0 | 0 | 0 | 0 | ++++ |
| Dobutamine (μg/kg/min) | | | | | | |
| 2–10 | + | 0 | ++++ | ++ | 0 | 0 |
| >10–20 | ++ | 0 | ++++ | +++ | 0 | 0 |

Activity ranges from no activity (0) to maximal activity (++++); ?, activity is unknown.
*Abbreviations:* DA, dopaminergic receptor; V, vasopressin receptor.

resuscitation when compared with the other catecholamine agents.[16] However, without adequate fluid resuscitation, norepinephrine may decrease perfusion to the gastric and renal systems. This again highlights the need for adequate fluid resuscitation.[16]

Dopamine should be initiated at a dose of 2 to 5 μg/kg/min and titrated to a maximum dose of 20 to 25 μg/kg/min. Dopamine has more beta agonist effects compared with norepinephrine and causes more tachyarrhythmias than norepinephrine.[16,29,30] Both agents are effective in restoring MAPs in patients who remain in shock after volume resuscitation. Low-dose dopamine to maintain renal function or to increase renal blood pressure has fallen out of favor, and recent data do not support its use for this indication (Grade 1A).[5,31,32]

Phenylephrine is generally considered one of the second-line agents, mainly because of the lack of available literature and possible adverse effects from the agent (Grade 2C).[5] Phenylephrine is a strong vasoconstrictor agent that has only alpha activity. Because of the lack of beta agonist effects, phenylephrine may be a good alternative in patients with underlying tachyarrhythmias. When used, phenylephrine increases MAPs at doses of 0.25 to 0.5 μg/kg/min. Although rarely needed clinically, phenylephrine may be titrated to a maximum dose of 8 μg/kg/min.[5] Phenylephrine has dose-dependent negative effects on the splanchnic blood flow.[5,33]

Epinephrine has beta and alpha agonist effects and until recently has been the last vasoconstrictor agent considered for use, mainly because of its negative effects on lactate and splanchnic perfusion. Some data suggest a decrease in splanchnic blood flow and increases in systemic and regional lactate concentrations.[5,34,35] However, newer studies do not support these data, and the current guidelines suggest using epinephrine as the agent of choice when the shock is poorly responsive to norepinephrine or dopamine (Grade 2B).[5,36] Epinephrine has been used in doses ranging from 0.01 to 0.5 μg/kg/min in patients with septic shock.[5,16,34,35]

Vasopressin has been used for more than 10 years for the management of vasodilatory shock.[37] Several investigators have described a relative vasopressin deficiency in patients with septic shock.[38,39] Since then, vasopressin has been used in low doses to help replenish this deficiency. Low-dose vasopressin can be considered after starting treatment with norepinephrine or other catecholamines (Grade 2C).[5] The Vasopressin and Septic Shock Trial investigators designed a multicentered, randomized study evaluating the effects of low-dose vasopressin when compared with norepinephrine. Vasopressin was started at a dose of 0.01 U/min and titrated to a maximum dose of 0.03 U/min. The investigators concluded that low-dose vasopressin did not reduce mortality in patients with septic shock, but it was as effective and safe compared with norepinephrine. In this study, vasopressin may have a benefit in outcomes in patients with lower dose of norepinephrine (<15 μg/min); however, this needs to be further studied.[40] In most cases, vasopressin is initiated at doses of 0.01 to 0.04 U/min. Doses greater than 0.04 U/min have been shown to cause more adverse cardiovascular effects (ischemia and/or arrhythmias) and should not be used routinely.[41] Compared with the catecholamine vasopressors, vasopressin has a much longer duration of action (approximate half-life of 2 and 10 minutes, respectively).[42,43] Because of the relative vasopressin deficiency in septic shock and the longer duration of action of vasopressin, it should be the last agent titrated off. After all catecholamine agents have been titrated off, vasopressin can be decreased by 25% every 30 to 60 minutes, while maintaining an adequate blood pressure. Vasopressin can decrease cardiac output and decrease splanchnic perfusion, and long-term outcome data are needed.[16,41,44–46] Also, because vasopressin is a potent vasoconstrictor, it should be administered through central venous access. There have been reports of ischemic extremities after the infiltration of vasopressin when administered through a peripheral vein.[47–49]

Dobutamine acts mainly on the beta receptors to increase cardiac contractility (beta-1 effects) and to decrease systemic vascular resistance (beta-2 effects). Dobutamine may be added when there is evidence or suspicion of myocardial dysfunction (Grade 1C); however, it should not be used to increase cardiac output beyond normal levels (Grade 1B).[5] The EGDT study administered dobutamine to patients with an Scvo$_2$ of less than 70% after transfusion therapy (Grade 2C).[5,14] Approximately 15% of patients with severe sepsis have myocardial dysfunction, making dobutamine therapy a valid option in patients with evidence of low cardiac output states.[14,16,30] Dobutamine is typically initiated at doses of 2.5 to 5 μg/kg/min and titrated every 5 to 10 minutes to a maximum of 20 μg/kg/min based on the percentage of Svo$_2$ or Scvo$_2$ or cardiac output.[5,16] Dobutamine can cause dose-related hypotension because of the beta-2 venous dilation effects. In those patients, a vasoconstrictor (eg, norepinephrine, phenylephrine, or dopamine) may be started to maintain optimal blood pressure. Dobutamine can also cause dose-related tachyarrhythmias from the beta-1 stimulation, which may limit its use in some patients.[16]

## CASE REVISITED

The patient was recognized to have septic shock (4 of the SIRS criteria, plus an infection and acute organ dysfunction, with failure to respond to fluid resuscitation). Goal-directed therapy was initiated, which included a CVP of 8 to 12 mm Hg, MAP of more than 65 mm Hg, and central venous oxygen saturation more than 70%. Initial resuscitation for septic shock was initiated with 1000 mL of crystalloids given over 20 minutes, which elevated his blood pressure to 92/48 mm Hg with a MAP of 62 mm Hg. Another 1000 mL bolus of crystalloids was ordered for continued fluid resuscitation. Within the first hour, broad-spectrum intravenous antibiotics and antifungals were initiated after blood cultures were obtained, one from a peripheral phlebotomy puncture and another from the central line. He was transferred to the ICU, and an arterial line was placed for continuous blood pressure monitoring. The central venous oxygen saturation was 65%. He remained hypotensive despite repeated fluid boluses, and a norepinephrine drip was initiated. A repeat serum lactate was 8 mg/dL. Two units of packed red blood cells were given, and a dobutamine drip was initiated. Preparations were made for an emergent exploratory surgery and washout for source control.

In the operating room, an anastomotic dehiscence was found and repaired. Postoperatively, the patient was transferred back to the ICU and remained intubated for ventilatory support. On the second postoperative day from the revision, the vasopressor and sedation were weaned off because his blood pressure stabilized and he was extubated. Blood cultures returned negative for bacterial growth; however, peritoneal fluid cultures obtained during the revision procedure revealed *Escherichia coli*, *Streptococcus* spp, and *Candida* spp. The patient completed a full course of intravenous antibiotics and had no further complications. He made a full recovery.

## SUMMARY

The postoperative or bedside nurse is usually the first health care member to observe the subtle initial changes a patient exhibits in early sepsis. As an infection develops into sepsis, the patient may have early mental status changes, hyper- or hypothermia, changes in skin color or temperature, hyperglycemia, and decreases in urine output. The gradual trend of vital sign changes and serum laboratory changes can also be identified by the astute bedside nurse. It is crucial to respond rapidly if sepsis is suspected, because delay in implementation of treatment can lead to acute organ failure and possibly death. Within the first hour of recognition of sepsis, laboratory samples and cultures should be obtained, fluid resuscitation should be initiated, and antibiotics should be administered. In addition to these primary interventions, transfer to an ICU should be coordinated if necessary and a potential source should be identified and addressed. To decrease mortality and morbidity, all these measures should be performed within 6 hours of presentation. Knowing the standards of early goal-directed therapy, early source control and antibiotics, and vasopressor effects can help the nurse anticipate the plan of care for the patient, expediting the treatments needed to stabilize and reverse the life-threatening progression of sepsis.

## REFERENCES

1. Martin GS, Mannino DM, Eaton S, et al. The epidemiology of sepsis in the United States from 1979 to 2000. N Engl J Med 2003;348:1546–54.
2. Angus DC, Linde-Zwirble WT, Lidicker J, et al. Epidemiology of severe sepsis in the United States: analysis of incidence, outcome, and associated costs of care. Crit Care Med 2001;29:1303–10.
3. Martin GS, Mannino DM, Moss M. The effect of age on the development and outcome of adult sepsis. Crit Care Med 2006;34:15–21.
4. Guidet B, Aegerter P, Gauzit R, et al. Incidence and impact of organ dysfunctions associated with sepsis. Chest 2005;127:942–51.
5. Dellinger RP, Levy MM, Carlet JM, et al. Surviving Sepsis Campaign: international guidelines for management of severe sepsis and septic shock: 2008. Crit Care Med 2008;36:296–327.

6. Nguyen HB, Corbett SW, Steele R, et al. Implementation of a bundle of quality indicators for the early management of severe sepsis and septic shock is associated with decreased mortality. Crit Care Med 2007;35:1105–12.

7. Ferrer R, Artigas A, Levy M, et al. Improvement in process of care and outcome after multicenter severe sepsis educational program in Spain. JAMA 2008;299:2294–303.

8. Bone RC, Balk R, Cerra FB, et al. ACCP/SCCM Consensus Conference: definitions for sepsis and organ failure and guidelines for use of innovative therapies in sepsis. Chest 1992;101:1644–55.

9. Novotny A, Emmanuel K, Matevossian E, et al. Use of procalcitonin for early prediction of lethal outcome of postoperative sepsis. Am J Surg 2007;194:35–9.

10. Muller B, Becker KL, Schachinger H, et al. Calcitonin precursors are reliable markers of sepsis in a medical intensive care unit. Crit Care Med 2000;28:977–83.

11. Becker KL, Snider R, Nylen ES. Procalcitonin assay in systemic inflammation, infection, and sepsis: clinical utility and limitations. Crit Care Med 2008;36:941–52.

12. Luzzani A, Polati E, Dorizzi R, et al. Comparison of procalcitonin and C-reactive protein as markers of sepsis. Crit Care Med 2003;31:1737–41.

13. Donnino MW, Nguyen B, Jacobsen G, et al. Cryptic septic shock: a sub-analysis of early, goal-directed therapy [abstract]. Chest 2003;124:90S.

14. Rivers E, Nguyen B, Havstad S, et al. Early goal-directed therapy in the treatment of severe sepsis and septic shock. N Engl J Med 2001;345:1368–77.

15. Otero RM, Nguyen B, Huang DT, et al. Early goal-directed therapy in severe sepsis and septic shock revisited. Concepts, controversies, and contemporary findings. Chest 2006;130:1579–95.

16. Hollenberg SM, Ahrens TS, Annane D, et al. Practice parameters for hemodynamic support of sepsis in adult patients: 2004 update. Crit Care Med 2004;32:1928–48.

17. Ahrens T. Hemodynamics in sepsis. AACN Adv Crit Care 2006;17:435–45.

18. Pinsky MR. Hemodynamic evaluation and monitoring in the ICU. Chest 2007;132:2020–9.

19. Finfer S, Bellomo R, Boyce N, et al. A comparison of albumin and saline for fluid resuscitation in the intensive care unit. N Engl J Med 2004;350:2247–56.

20. American Thoracic Society. Evidence-based colloid use in the critically ill: American Thoracic Society Consensus Statement. Am J Respir Crit Care Med 2004;170:1247–59.

21. Ernest D, Belzberg AS, Dodek PM. Distribution of normal saline and 5% albumin infusions in septic patients. Crit Care Med 1999;27:46–50.

22. Wiedemann HP, Wheeler AP, Bernard GR, et al. Comparison of two fluid-management strategies in acute lung injury. N Engl J Med 2006;354:2564–75.

23. Kumar A, Roberts D, Wood KE, et al. Duration of hypotension before initiation of effective antimicrobial therapy is the critical determinant of survival in human septic shock. Crit Care Med 2006;34:1589–96.

24. Ferrer R, Artigas A, Suarez D, et al. Effectiveness of treatments in severe sepsis: a prospective multicenter observational study. Am J Respir Crit Care Med 2009;180:861–6.

25. Morrell M, Fraser VJ, Kollef MH. Delaying the empiric treatment of candida bloodstream infection until positive blood culture results are obtained: a potential risk factor for hospital mortality. Antimicrob Agents Chemother 2005;49:3640–5.

26. Chastre J, Wolff M, Fagon JY, et al. Comparison of 8 versus 15 days of antibiotic therapy for ventilator-associated pneumonia in adults: a randomized trial. JAMA 2003;290:2588–98.

27. Moss RL, Musemeche CA, Kosloske AM. Necrotizing fasciitis in children: prompt recognition and aggressive therapy improve survival. J Pediatr Surg 1996;31(8): 1142–6.
28. Kumar A, Wood K, Gurka D, et al. Outcome of septic shock correlates with duration of hypotension prior to source control implementation. Abstr Intersci Conf Antimicrob Agents Chemother Intersci Conf Antimicrob Agents Chemother 2004;350:K-1222.
29. Regnier B, Rapin M, Gory G, et al. Haemodynamic effects of dopamine in septic shock. Intensive Care Med 1977;3:47–53.
30. Dellinger RP. Cardiovascular management of septic shock. Crit Care Med 2003; 31:946–55.
31. Schenarts PJ, Sagraves SG, Bard MR, et al. Low-dose dopamine: a physiologically based review. Curr Surg 2006;63:219–25.
32. Bellomo R, Chapman M, Finfer S, et al. Low-dose dopamine in patients with early renal dysfunction: a placebo-controlled randomized trial. Lancet 2000;356: 2139–43.
33. Morelli A, Lange M, Ertmer C, et al. Short-term effects of phenylephrine on systemic and regional hemodynamics in patients with septic shock: a crossover pilot study. Shock 2008;29:446–51.
34. Levy B, Bollaert PE, Charpentier C, et al. Comparison of norepinephrine and dobutamine to epinephrine for hemodynamics, lactate metabolism, and gastric tonometric variables in septic shock: a prospective, randomised study. Intensive Care Med 1997;23:282–7.
35. Myburgh JA, Higgins A, Jovanovska A, et al. A comparison of epinephrine and norepinephrine in critically ill patients. Intensive Care Med 2008;34: 2226–34.
36. Annane D, Vignon P, Renault A, et al. Norepinephrine plus dobutamine versus epinephrine alone for management of septic shock: a randomised trial. Lancet 2007;370:676–84.
37. Landry DW, Levin HR, Gallant EM, et al. Vasopressin pressor hypersensitivity in vasodilatory septic shock. Crit Care Med 1997;25:1279–82.
38. Sharshar T, Carlier R, Blanchard A, et al. Depletion of neurohypophyseal content of vasopressin in septic shock. Crit Care Med 2002;30:497–500.
39. Sharshar T, Blanchard A, Paillard M, et al. Circulating vasopressin levels in septic shock. Crit Care Med 2003;31:1752–8.
40. Russell JA, Walley KR, Singer J, et al. Vasopressin versus norepinephrine infusion in patients with septic shock. N Engl J Med 2008;358:877–87.
41. Holmes CL, Patel BM, Russell JA, et al. Physiology of vasopressin relevant to management of septic shock. Chest 2001;120:989–1002.
42. Czaczkes JW, Kleeman CR, Koenig M. Physiologic studies of antidiuretic hormone by its direct measurement in human plasma. J Clin Invest 1964;43: 1625–40.
43. Beloeil H, Mazoit JX, Benhamou D, et al. Norepinephrine kinetics and dynamics in septic shock and trauma patients. Br J Anaesth 2005;95:782–8.
44. Leone M, Martin C. Vasopressor use in septic shock. Curr Opin Anaesthesiol 2008;21:141–7.
45. Russell JA. Vasopressin use in septic shock. Crit Care Med 2007;35:S609–15.
46. Hauser B, Asfar P, Calzia E, et al. Vasopressin in vasodilatory shock: is the heart in danger? Crit Care 2008;12:132.
47. Bunker N, Higgins D. Peripheral administration of vasopressin for catecholamine-resistant hypotension complicated by skin necrosis. Crit Care Med 2006;34:935.

48. Kahn JM, Kress JP, Hall JB. Skin necrosis after extravasation of low-dose vaso-pressin administered for septic shock. Crit Care Med 2002;30:1899–901.
49. Dunser MW, Mayr AJ, Tur A, et al. Ischemic skin lesions as a complication of continuous vasopressin infusion in catecholamine-resistant vasodilatory shock: incidence and risk factors. Crit Care Med 2003;31:1394–8.

# Local Anesthetic Use in Perioperative Areas

Carolyn J. Friel, RPh, PhD[a],*, Carol Eliadi, APRN, EdD, JD[b],
Kimberly A. Pesaturo, PharmD, BCPS[c]

**KEYWORDS**

- Anesthesia • Lidocaine • Local anesthesia
- Lidocaine with epinephrine
- Local anesthetic toxicity • Local anesthetic overdose

Local anesthesia is a pharmacologic technique used to render a small part of the body insensitive to pain. It allows the patient to safely undergo select medical or surgical procedures with reduced pain without altering level of consciousness. Regional anesthesia, including epidural and spinal anesthesia, and general anesthesia are aimed at anesthetizing a larger part of the body or the total body. Surface anesthesia involves the application of a local anesthetic spray, solution, or cream to the skin or to a mucous membrane. The effect is short-lasting and is limited to the area of contact by the pharmacologic agent. Infiltration anesthesia involves the injection of a local anesthetic agent into the tissue to be anesthetized. This article addresses local anesthesia and covers surface and infiltration anesthesia.

The perioperative nurse is responsible for monitoring patients receiving local anesthetics, which are used throughout the preoperative, intraoperative, and postoperative phases of surgery. Due to cost savings, reduced time in postoperative settings, and improved safety profiles over general anesthetics, more procedures are now routinely done under local anesthesia.[1–4] For example, laser surgery,[5] biopsies,[6] inguinal hernia repairs,[7] laparoscopic procedures,[1,8] and thoracoscopic procedures[9] may now occur with local anesthetics as the primary medication for pain management. Local anesthesia may also be used before venous cannulation, lumbar puncture, or skin suturing, or it may be used to prevent pain caused by bone and/or muscle manipulations. This article reviews the physiology of pain, the mechanism of action and chemistry of the local anesthetics, adverse reactions,

[a] Department of Pharmaceutical Sciences, School of Pharmacy, Massachusetts College of Pharmacy and Health Sciences-Worcester, 19 Foster Street, Worcester, MA 01608, USA
[b] Department of Nursing, School of Nursing, Massachusetts College of Pharmacy and Health Sciences-Worcester, 25 Foster Street, Worcester, MA 01608, USA
[c] Department of Pharmacy Practice, School of Pharmacy, Massachusetts College of Pharmacy and Health Sciences-Worcester, 19 Foster Street, Worcester, MA 01608, USA
* Corresponding author.
*E-mail address:* carolyn.friel@mcphs.edu

Perioperative Nursing Clinics 5 (2010) 203–214
doi:10.1016/j.cpen.2010.02.001
1556-7931/10/$ – see front matter © 2010 Elsevier Inc. All rights reserved.

common dosages, and special considerations for the perioperative nurse managing patients receiving local anesthetics.

## PHYSIOLOGY OF PAIN

Pain is perceived by the brain when a nerve cell, a neuron, transmits the message via an action potential that originates at the site of the origin of pain. Local anesthetics block both the generation of the action potential and the conduction of the action potential along the nerve. By blocking the action potential, the signal is not received by the brain and the patient does not perceive pain. Because local anesthetics block both the generation of the impulse and the propagation of the action potential, they can be used prophylactically or to treat acute pain in the perioperative setting.

A resting neuron has an interior electrical potential of −70 mV that results from the different concentration of ions on the inside and outside of the neuronal membrane. To generate an action potential, the electrical potential in the interior of the neuron must first be increased to around −55 mV. This initial depolarization is the result of an inward flow of positively charged sodium ions through the sodium channel. When the −55 mV firing threshold is reached, the permeability of the membrane to sodium further increases and massive amounts of sodium ions flow into the cell, leaving the cell depolarized. The depolarization along one part of the axon creates depolarization along the neighboring sections of the membrane, and the electrical message moves along the axon toward the central nervous system (CNS) sending the "message of pain" to the brain (**Fig. 1A**).[10]

Nerve cells that carry messages from the brain to the periphery are called motor neurons or efferent nerves. Nerve cells that transmit messages from the periphery to the CNS are sensory neurons or afferent nerves. Local anesthetics have varying effects on all nerve cells depending on the diameter of the nerve fiber, myelination, firing rate, and location of the nerve. Smaller-diameter nerve fibers are affected more than larger ones. In general, myelinated nerve cells, those that contain a myelin sheath interspersed along the axon, are blocked by local anesthetics before unmyelinated nerves. Nerve fibers that are actively firing are blocked by local anesthetics faster than those that are not firing. In general, nerve fibers that mediate pain and temperature sensation are more susceptible to local anesthetics than those that mediate touch, pressure, and motor information.[11]

## MECHANISM OF ACTION OF LOCAL ANESTHETICS

The local anesthetics work by blocking the flow of sodium ions into the neuron. After injection or absorption through the skin, the local anesthetic equilibrates between its positively charged form and a neutral form. The amount of drug that is in the neutral form is important. It is the neutral form of the drug that penetrates the lipophilic nerve membrane and can have a biologic effect (see the section "Chemistry of the local anesthetics").[12,13] Once the drug is inside the nerve it reequilibrates and now the cationic (positively charged) form of the drug binds to the local anesthetic binding site on the sodium channel. When the anesthetic drug is bound to the sodium channel it blocks the passage of sodium ions through the channel (see **Fig. 1**B). By preventing sodium ions from entering the neuron, the cell cannot depolarize and no "pain message" is sent along the axon to the brain.

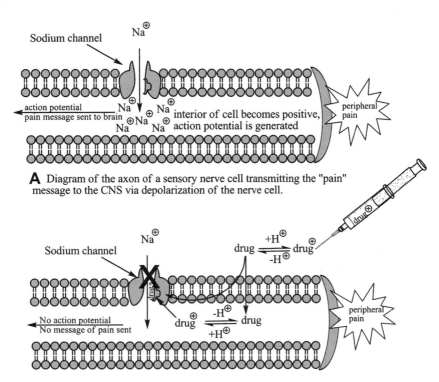

**A** Diagram of the axon of a sensory nerve cell transmitting the "pain" message to the CNS via depolarization of the nerve cell.

**B** Local anesthetic drugs, in their ionized form, bind to the sodium channel and prevent sodium from entering the nerve cell. The action potential is thus blocked and the message of pain is not sent to the brain.

**Fig. 1.** Mechanism of action of local anesthetics. (*A*) Axon of a sensory nerve cell transmits the "pain message" to the CNS via depolarization of the nerve cell. (*B*) Local anesthetic drugs, in their ionized form, bind to the sodium channel and prevent sodium from entering the nerve cell. The action potential is thus blocked and the message of pain is not sent to the brain.

## CHEMISTRY OF THE LOCAL ANESTHETICS

Most local anesthetics are composed of a lipophilic (fat-loving) aromatic ring, a linking group that contains either an ester or an amide and a hydrophilic (water-soluble) nitrogen group capable of binding hydrogen and becoming charged (**Fig. 2**). Most local anesthetics have a pKa around physiologic pH; so on injection the drug is found in both its cationic (+) and its neutral state.[14] The ionization state of the drug plays a considerable role in the onset of action. Local anesthetics are formulated by the manufacturer in an acidic pH, and thus the drug is charged in the vial. The acidic formulation provides water solubility to the drug and prevents it from precipitating out in the vial. The acidic formulation presents two clinical problems for the nurse practitioner administering the drug. First, charged compounds do not penetrate membranes or intact skin well and must be injected into the affected area. The charged form of the drug must first dissociate to the uncharged form, cross the nerve membrane, reequilibrate with its charged form, and then bind to the local anesthetic binding site on the sodium channel (see **Fig. 1**B). The amount of drug that can dissociate into the neutral form and thus penetrate the nerve membrane is a function of the pH of the tissue. Infected tissue is known to have a more acidic pH, and thus less drug

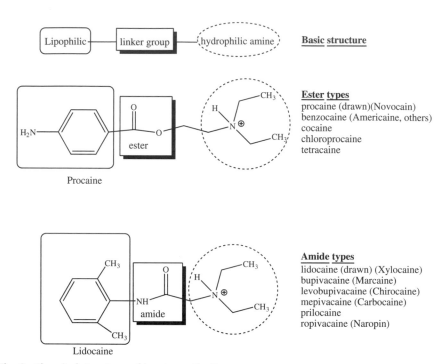

**Fig. 2.** Chemical structure of local anesthetics.

will be in the neutral form; therefore less drug will penetrate the nerve membrane. Infected tissue may therefore require larger doses of anesthetic drug to produce the same level of anesthesia. The second problem that the acidic formulation of the drug offers is that it is painful on injection. Because the anesthetic is used to decrease pain, this is an unwelcome problem. Publications exist that condone the addition of sodium bicarbonate to the anesthetic vial to decrease the acidity, decrease the pain on injection, and possibly hasten the onset of action by increasing the membrane permeable neutral form of the drug.[15–18] Care must be taken to follow published guidelines, because overzealous use of sodium bicarbonate causes the drug to precipitate out in the vial.

## LOCAL ANESTHETICS WITH VASOCONSTRICTORS

The duration of the local anesthetic action depends on the period of time it resides on the local anesthetic binding site, blocking the action potential. To increase the residence time at the site of injection, local anesthetics are available in combination with vasoconstrictors such as epinephrine, levonordefrin, and phenylephrine (**Table 1**). Vasoconstrictors constrict blood vessels, decreasing blood flow at the site of administration; this effect can be observed as skin mottling or blanching. The reduced perfusion at the site of administration allows more local anesthetic to stay at the applied site resulting in decreased systemic absorption. For example, 400 mg of lidocaine without a vasoconstrictor infiltrated in the oral cavity results in a peak plasma level of 4.3 μg/mL, whereas a 400-mg dose of lidocaine with a vasoconstrictor yields a peak plasma level of only 3.0 μg/mL.[10] The decreased blood perfusion also reduces the amount of metabolizing enzymes present at the site of administration, which also contributes to the extended duration of action of local anesthetics with vasoconstrictors when compared with local anesthetics without vasoconstrictors. By constricting the local capillary bed, vasoconstrictors also reduce bleeding, and this can be advantageous during surgical procedures.

According to the manufacturer, anesthetics with a vasoconstrictor should be used with caution in areas of the body supplied by end arteries, such as the fingers and toes,[19] although there is mounting evidence that excluding vasoconstrictors in these situations is unwarranted.[20] Local anesthetics with vasoconstrictors should also be used with caution in patients with preexisting cardiovascular or thyroid disease. Studies have shown that an injection (oral cavity) of anesthetic with as little as 20 µg of epinephrine caused a small but significant increase in heart rate.[21,22] The side effects of the absorbed epinephrine must therefore be weighed against the increased dose of local anesthetic that would otherwise be required.

The perioperative nurse must know the maximum recommended dose of the local anesthetic, reviewed by Ivey,[23] as well as how to calculate the amount of vasoconstrictor the patient is receiving. The amount of vasoconstrictor present in the local anesthetic solution is given as a ratio. For example, a lidocaine injection with vasoconstrictor 1:100,000 means that the solution contains 1 g of vasoconstrictor for every 100,000 mL of solution. Therefore, a 1:100,000 ratio contains 1000 mg/100,000 mL or 0.01 mg/mL of vasoconstrictor. Maximum recommended doses of vasoconstrictors are often represented in microgram (µg) quantities (1 mg = 1000 µg). Therefore, a 1:100,000 ratio contains 10 µg/mL of vasoconstrictor. A patient who receives 12.5 mL of anesthetic with 1:100,000 epinephrine has received 125 µg of epinephrine. Using the same conversions, an anesthetic solution with 1:200,000 epinephrine contains 1 g/200,000 mL or 0.005 mg/mL or 5 µg/mL. Therefore, 12.5 mL of anesthetic with 1:200,000 epinephrine contains 62.5 µg of epinephrine.

## ADVERSE REACTIONS

Adverse reactions to local anesthetics include hypersensitivity reactions and toxicity reactions. The perioperative nurse should be familiar with these potential adverse reactions and should recognize the signs and symptoms of each. The emergency management of each type of adverse reaction is different and discussed in the following sections.

### Hypersensitivity Reactions

Allergic reactions to local anesthetics are rare.[24] The perioperative nurse should recognize that allergic reactions to local anesthetics are not dose dependent and may occur even when using less than the recommended maximum dose. Allergic reactions to any drug results in immune-mediated manifestations that may include bronchospasms, urticaria, fever, dermatitis, photosensitivity, and anaphylaxis.[10] A patient receiving a local anesthetic may have an allergic reaction to the drug, a metabolite of the drug, the preservative, or any other additive in the drug preparation. Most local anesthetic allergic reactions are due to the ester type local anesthetics (see **Fig. 2**). A patient with a history of an allergic reaction to any ester anesthetic should not receive any local anesthetic from this class. All ester anesthetics are metabolized to para-aminobenzoic acid (PABA) (**Fig. 3**), which is thought to be the hapten responsible for immune-mediated allergic reactions.[24] Patients who are allergic to ester anesthetics must also not receive any drug that uses a methylparaben preservative. Methylparaben and its metabolites are chemically similar to PABA, and crossover sensitivity reactions are possible. Therefore, patients with an allergic reaction to any

**Table 1**
Common medications used for local anesthesia in the adult perioperative setting

| Product | Dosage Forms Available | Typical Dose/Route | Maximum Dose | Time to Onset | Duration of Effect | Special Considerations |
|---|---|---|---|---|---|---|
| Topical creams, gels, and viscous formulations | | | | | | |
| 2.5% Prilocaine, 2.5% lidocaine[41,42] | Cream; self-adhesive disc (contains 1 g total product) | Apply thick layer to intact skin or 1–2 g cream over 10 cm$^2$ intact skin (or apply 1 disc) | 20 g over 200 cm$^2$ skin surface for no more than 4 h | 1–2 h | Peak effect for 2–3 h with duration of 1–2 h after removal | Cream should be covered with occlusive dressing |
| Topical lidocaine, various concentrations[41] | Cream/gel/jelly | Apply thin layer to intact skin up to 3 times/day as needed | Varies; gel: 4.5 mg/kg up to a maximum of 300 mg; do not leave on for >2 h | 20–30 min | 10 min–1 h | Remove cream and clean area before procedure; avoid application to mucous membranes |
| 2% Lidocaine viscous[41,43] | 20 mg/mL topical solution | 5–10 mL (100–200 mg) swish/spit or swish/swallow for painful mucous membranes; 10–15 mL (200–300 mg) before instrumentation of upper respiratory tract | 6 doses/24 h; do not exceed 60 mL (1200 mg)/24 h Do not exceed 20 mL (400 mg) in a single dose | 5 min | 10–20 min | Ineffective on application to intact skin |
| Benzocaine spray[41,44] | 20% aerosol oral spray | Hold extension tube 1–2 in from area and spray for half a second | 2 consecutive half-a-second sprays; use only every 6 h | 30–60 s | 12–15 min | Methemoglobinemia reported after overdose; suppresses gag reflex if swallowed |

| Drug | Formulation | Dose/Application | Maximum Dose | Onset | Duration | Notes |
|---|---|---|---|---|---|---|
| Cocaine[41] | 4% and 10% topical solution | 1%–4% applied topically to mucosa; use lowest dose possible to produce effect | 10% solution or 1 mg/kg (up to 200 mg) | 1–5 min | 30 min or greater (dose-dependent) | For topical use only |
| **Injectable local anesthetics with or without adjunct vasoconstrictors** | | | | | | |
| Lidocaine hydrochloride[26,41] | 0.5%–2% solution for injection | Up to 400 mg/dose for local infiltration | 4.5 mg/kg or 400 mg/ single dose; do not repeat within 2 h | 45–90 s | 1–3 h | May be administered with 1:50,000, 1:200,000, or 1:100,000 epinephrine[a] |
| Procaine[41,45] | 1%, 2% injectible solution | 0.25%–0.5% for local infiltration or 350–600 mg/single dose | 1000 mg per single dose | 2–5 min | 1 h | May be administered with 1:200,000 or 1:100,000 epinephrine[a] |
| Bupivacaine[41] | 0.25%, 0.5%, 0.75% injectible solution | 0.25% for local infiltration | 175 mg for infiltration | 4–10 min | 2–9 h | May be administered with 1:200,000 or 1:100,000 epinephrine[a] |
| Levobupivacaine[41,46] | 2.5 or 5 mg/mL injectible solution | 0.25% for local infiltration or 150 mg/single dose | 695 mg in 24 h | 6–10 min | 1–8 h | |
| Ropivacaine[41,47] | 2, 5, 7.5, 10 mg/mL injectible solution | 1–40 mL of 0.5% or 1–100 mL of 0.2% for local infiltration or 200 mg/single dose | 300 mg | 3–15 min | 2–6 h | |
| Mepivacaine[41,48] | 1%, 1.5%, 2%, and 3% | 180 mg/single dose for local infiltration use 0.5% to 1% solution | 400 mg | 7–15 min | 2–2.5 h | May be administered with levonordefrin 1:20,000 |

[a] Epinephrine dose should not exceed 3 μg/kg or 0.2 mg per dental appointment.
*Data from* Lacy CF, Armstrong LL, Goldman MP, et al, editors. Drug information handbook. Hudson (OH): Lexi-Comp Inc; 2005.

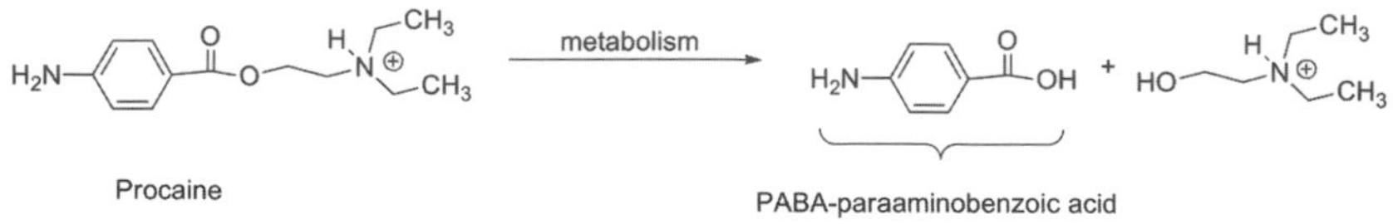

Fig. 3. Metabolism of procaine to PABA.

ester anesthetic may use an amide type local anesthetic as long as methylparaben is not the preservative used.

An additional allergy history that nurses must be aware of is to sulfites (not sulfa drugs). Metabisulfites are used to extend the shelf life in many food products, creams, and medications, including some local anesthetics with vasoconstrictors.[25] The overall risk of sulfite allergies in the general population is not known but it is believed to be higher in patients with asthma.[26] Allergic manifestations to metabisulfites include asthmatic symptoms and may progress to anaphylactic reactions.

Treatment of allergic reactions begins by discontinuing the offending agent. Supportive therapy with drugs such as epinephrine, antihistamines, and systemic corticosteroids follows, depending on the severity of the symptoms.[27]

## Toxicity Reactions

### Overdoses

Overdoses result when the systemic absorption of the drug is high enough to cause adverse reactions in an organ or tissue. Elevated blood levels may result from exceeding the maximum recommended dose, because overdose reactions are dose dependent. **Table 1** lists typical doses and the maximum recommended dose for some common local anesthetics. The clinician should keep in mind that the required dose for any local anesthetic varies with the anesthetic procedure, the vascularity of the tissue, the area to be anesthetized, and the duration of the desired effect. The recommended dose is always the smallest dose required to provide comfort during the specific procedure. Overdoses may occur due to inadvertent intravascular administration or even absorption from excessive topical applications.[28,29] Overdose reactions may also occur in patients with preexisting conditions, even if the maximum recommended dose is not exceeded. Patients with hepatic disease, resulting in reduced metabolism of the drug, or patients with renal disease, resulting in reduced elimination of the drug, may experience elevated drug blood levels. Signs of local anesthetic overdose (in progressive order) include talkativeness, excitability, slurred speech, stutter, euphoria, dysarthria, nystagmus, sweating, vomiting, disorientation, elevated blood pressure, elevated heart rate, elevated respiratory rate, tonic-clonic seizure, generalized CNS depression, depressed blood pressure, depressed heart rate, depressed respiratory rate, coma, and death.[10]

Treatment of local anesthetic overdoses depends on the severity of the overdose. Mild cases may require no specific treatment after discontinuing the administration of the drug. Severe reactions necessitate basic emergency management and the Association of Operating Room Nurses (AORN) guidelines recommend that at a minimum, available personnel should be competent in basic life support.[30] Treatment of severe overdose reactions may require the administration of oxygen, anticonvulsants, and vasopressors. In severe overdose situations, protocols for treatment include the intravascular infusion of a lipid emulsion.[29,31] The lipid emulsion acts as a "drug sink" for the local anesthetic molecule, and multiple case reports support its use to treat local anesthetic overdoses.[32–34]

*Methemoglobinemia*

Methemoglobinemia results when the hemoglobin in red blood cells is oxidized by a drug or drug metabolite and loses its ability to carry oxygen. This can be caused by many drugs including lidocaine,[35] prilocaine,[36] and benzocaine.[37] When the concentration of methemoglobin is greater than 30% (normal level = 1%) symptoms such as dizziness, headache, tachycardia, and weakness develop. When the concentration is greater than 45% cardiac arrhythmias, metabolic acidosis, hypoxia, seizures, and coma may occur. Concentrations above 70% are rapidly fatal.[38] The clinical indicator often leading to the diagnosis of methemoglobinemia is cyanosis that does not respond to treatment with 100% oxygen. Treatment includes standard supportive measures and an intravenous infusion of 1% methylene blue solution (1–2 mg/kg) for 5 minutes.[38]

## IMPLICATIONS FOR NURSING PRACTICE

The AORN has published recommended practices for monitoring the patient receiving local anesthesia.[30] The perioperative nurse is thus referred to these guidelines to read the full set of nine recommended practices. These recommendations include a preoperative assessment and development of an individualized plan of care. The preoperative assessment should include a detailed allergy history including reactions to prior local anesthetics, PABA, methylparaben, or sulfites (Recommended Practice I). The AORN guidelines state that the perioperative registered nurse should be knowledgeable about medication administration and be able to recognize both desired responses and adverse reactions to anesthetic medications. See **Table 1** for information on commonly used local anesthetic agents. The "Adverse reaction" section of this article also includes how to identify the unique signs, symptoms, and treatments of methemoglobinemia, overdose and hypersensitivity reactions resulting from local anesthetic use. An additional AORN recommended practice states that the perioperative nurse should monitor and interpret the patient's physiologic and psychological responses throughout the procedure and before discharge. As discussed earlier, physiologic changes such as heart rate and level of consciousness as well as behavioral changes such as slurred speech or drowsiness require prompt intervention. Recommended Practice III states that "emergency medications, a source of supplemental oxygen, suction apparatus, resuscitative equipment, and qualified personnel should be readily available."[30]

Documentation of drug dosages, route, time, and effect are also part of the AORN recommended practices as well as legally and professionally important for communication when the patient transitions from perioperative care. Documentation of local anesthetics should clearly convey the dose of the local anesthetic as well as the vasoconstrictor given (see "Local anesthetics with vasoconstrictors" for calculation examples). Local anesthetics should not be left at the bedside, because this can promote inappropriate patient use and undocumented administration.

In addition to the recommended guidelines published by AORN, the perioperative nurse should adhere to the fundamental practices related to safe medication administration.[39] These include correctly identifying the patient. One of the Joint Commission's National Patient Safety Goals is to improve the accuracy of patient identification.[40] To achieve this safety goal, the Joint Commission requires a nurse to use at least two patient identifiers whenever administering medication. Neither identifier can be the patient's room number. Appropriate identifiers such as the person's name, medical record number, telephone number, photograph, or other person-specific identifier can be used. Before administering the local anesthetic, the nurse should read the physician's order carefully. Verbal orders should be read back to the prescriber and recorded in the medical record.[40] Although the nurse may apply many of the topical anesthetic agents, most local anesthetic agents are administered parenterally by the physician, dentist, surgeon, physician assistant, or nurse practitioner. Gloves should be worn by the practitioner while administering local anesthesia, and the lowest dose of anesthetic possible should be applied to the smallest area possible. After the administration of local anesthesia, the nurse should comfortably position the patient, assist patient movement when necessary, and prevent activities during which the patient might inflict unintentional personal harm.

## SUMMARY

The overall goal of local anesthesia is to provide a reduction or elimination of pain associated with local procedures. This article supplements the published AORN recommended practices for managing the patient receiving local anesthesia.[30] The physiology of pain is briefly reviewed to give the perioperative nurse a sound background for understanding the pharmacologic mechanism by which local anesthetics exert their action. The chemical classification of local anesthetics is included to help the clinician choose an anesthetic when patients have exhibited prior allergic reactions to one class of drugs. The signs and symptoms of local anesthetic adverse reactions are reviewed to help the perioperative nurse recognize the different presentations and managements of methemoglobinemia, overdose, and hypersensitivity reactions. Recognizing the potential seriousness of medication errors in the perioperative setting, safe medication administration fundamentals are reviewed to ensure that perioperative nurses adhere to hospital-wide medication administration policies.

## REFERENCES

1. Lipscomb GH, Dell JR, Ling FW, et al. A comparison of the cost of local versus general anesthesia for laparoscopic sterilization in an operating room setting. J Am Assoc Gynecol Laparosc 1996;3(2):277–81.
2. Trieshmann HW. Knee arthroscopy: a cost analysis of general and local anesthesia. Arthroscopy 1996;12(1):60–3.
3. Kehlet H, White PF. Optimizing anesthesia for inguinal herniorrhaphy: general, regional, or local anesthesia? Anesth Analg 2001;93(6):1367–9.
4. White PF, Kehlet H, Neal JM, et al. The role of the anesthesiologist in fast-track surgery: from multimodal analgesia to perioperative medical care. Anesth Analg 2007;104(6):1380–96.
5. Zeitels SM, Burns JA. Office-based laryngeal laser surgery with local anesthesia. Curr Opin Otolaryngol Head Neck Surg 2007;15(3):141–7.
6. Alavi AS, Soloway MS, Vaidya A, et al. Local anesthesia for ultrasound guided prostate biopsy: a prospective randomized trial comparing 2 methods. J Urol 2001;166(4):1343–5.
7. Peiper C, Tons C, Schippers E, et al. Local versus general anesthesia for Shouldice repair of the inguinal hernia. World J Surg 1994;18(6):912–5 [discussion: 915–6].
8. Bordahl PE, Raeder JC, Nordentoft J, et al. Laparoscopic sterilization under local or general anesthesia? A randomized study. Obstet Gynecol 1993;81(1):137–41.
9. Hatz RA, Kaps MF, Meimarakis G, et al. Long-term results after video-assisted thoracoscopic surgery for first-time and recurrent spontaneous pneumothorax. Ann Thorac Surg 2000;70(1):253–7.
10. Malamed S. Handbook of local anesthesia. St. Louis (MO): C.V. Mosby; 2004.

11. Catterall WA. From ionic currents to molecular mechanisms: the structure and function of voltage-gated sodium channels. Neuron 2000;26:13–25.
12. Hille B. Local anesthetics: hydrophilic and hydrophobic pathways for the drug-receptor reaction. J Gen Physiol 1977;69:497–515.
13. Strichartz G, Sanchez V, Arthur G, et al. Fundamental properties of local anesthetics. II. Measured octanol:buffer partition coefficients and pKa values of clinically used drugs. Anesth Analg 1990;71(2):158–70.
14. Lu M. Inhibitors of nerve conduction: local anesthetics. In: Lemke T, Williams D, Roche V, et al, editors. Foye's principle of medicinal chemistry. 6th edition. New York: Wolters Kluwer, Lippincott, Williams and Wilkins; 2008. p. 462.
15. Brogan J, Gerard X, Giarrusso E, et al. Comparison of plain, warmed, and buffered lidocaine for anesthesia of traumatic wounds. Ann Emerg Med 1995;26(2):121–5.
16. Wong D, Pawero CL. Reducing the pain of lidocaine. Am J Nurs 1997;97(1):17–8.
17. Li J, Brainard D. Premixed buffered lidocaine retains efficacy after prolonged room temperature storage. Am J Emerg Med 2000;18(2):235–6.
18. Sinnott CJ, Garfield JM, Thalhammer JG, et al. Addition of sodium bicarbonate to lidocaine decreases the duration of peripheral nerve block in the rat. Anesthesiology 2000;93(4):1045–52.
19. Lignospan (lidocaine hydrochloride and epinephrine for injection) [package insert]. New Castle (DE): Septodont; 2006.
20. Newman DH. Truth and epinephrine at our fingertips: unveiling the pseudoaxioms. Ann Emerg Med 2007;50(4):476–7.
21. Knoll-Kohler E, Frie A, Becker J, et al. Changes in plasma epinephrine concentration after dental infiltration anesthesia with different doses of epinephrine. Journal of Dental Research 1989;68(6):1098–101.
22. Tolas A, Pflug A, I lalter J. Arterial plasma epinephrine concentrations and hemodynamic responses after dental injection of local anesthetic with epinephrine. J Am Dent Assoc 1982;104(1):41–3.
23. Ivey DF. Local anesthesia. Implications for the perioperative nurse. AORN J 1987;45(3):682–9.
24. Eggleston ST, Lush LW. Understanding allergic reactions to local anesthetics. Ann Pharmacother 1996;30(7–8):851–7.
25. Finucane BT. Allergies to local anesthetics - the real truth. Can J Anaesth 2003;50(9):869–74.
26. Xylocaine (lidocaine hydrochloride injection) [package insert]. Wilmington (DE): AstraZeneca; 2008.
27. Riedl MA, Casillas AM. Adverse drug reactions: types and treatment options. Am Fam Physician 2003;68(9):1781–90.
28. Ukens C. Coed death tied to compounded drug (May). Drug Topics 2005. Available at: Drugtopics.com. Accessed February 18, 2010.
29. Turner-Lawrence DE, Kerns Ii W. Intravenous fat emulsion: a potential novel antidote. J Med Toxicol 2008;4(2):109–14.
30. AORN Recommended Practices Committee. Recommended practices for managing the patient receiving local anesthesia. AORN J 2007;85(5):965–71.
31. Weinberg G. Available at: lipidrescue.org. 2009. Accessed April 6, 2009.
32. Picard J, Meek T. Lipid emulsion to treat overdose of local anaesthetic: the gift of the glob. Anaesthesia 2006;61(2):107–9.
33. Rosenblatt MA, Abel M, Fischer GW, et al. Successful use of a 20% lipid emulsion to resuscitate a patient after a presumed bupivacaine-related cardiac arrest. Anesthesiology 2006;105(1):217–8.

34. Foxall G, McCahon R, Lamb J, et al. Levobupivacaine-induced seizures and cardiovascular collapse treated with Intralipid. Anaesthesia 2007;62(5):516–8.
35. Karim A, Ahmed S, Siddiqui R, et al. Methemoglobinemia complicating topical lidocaine used during endoscopic procedures. Am J Med 2001;111(2):150–3.
36. Kaendler L, Dorszewski A, Daehnert I. Methaemoglobinaemia after cardiac catheterisation: a rare cause of cyanosis. Heart 2004;90(9):e51.
37. Moore T, Walsh C, Cohen M. Reported adverse event cases of methemoglobinemia associated with benzocaine products. Arch Intern Med 2004;164(11): 1192–6.
38. Hegedus F, Herb K. Benzocaine-induced methemoglobinemia. Anesth Prog 2005;52(4):136–9.
39. Berman A, editor. Kozier and Erb's fundamentals of nursing: concepts, process, and practice. Upper Saddle River (NJ): Pearson Education, Inc; 2008. p. 848–50.
40. National Patient Safety Goals Performance Detail. Available at: http://www. jointcommissionreport.org/ safetyperformance/national-patient-safety-goals.aspx; 2009. Accessed April 8, 2009.
41. Lacy CF, Armstrong LL, Goldman MP, et al, editors. Drug information handbook. Hudson (OH): Lexi-Comp Inc; 2005. p. 183–1341.
42. EMLA (2.5% prilocaine and 2.5% lidocaine) [package insert]. Wilmington (DE): AstraZeneca; 2006.
43. Xylocaine Viscous 2% (lidocaine hydrochloride solution) [package insert]. Wilmington (DE): AstraZeneca; 2006.
44. Hurricaine Spray (20% benzocaine oral anesthetic) [package insert]. Waukegan (IL): Beutlich Pharmaceuticals; 2009.
45. Novocain (procaine hydrochloride) [package insert]. Lake Forest (IL): Hospira Inc; 2004.
46. Burlacu CL, Buggy DJ. Update on local anesthetics: focus on levobupivacaine. Ther Clin Risk Manag 2008;4(2):381–92.
47. Naropin (ropivacaine hydrochloride) [package insert]. Wilmington (DE): AstraZeneca; 2006.
48. Mepivacaine. Hudson (OH). Available at: http://www.crlonline.com. Lexi-Comp Online. Accessed May 30, 2009.

# Hybrid Interventional Radiology

Barry T. Katzen, MD[a], Jane Kiah, RN, MS[a],*,
Debbie Smith, RN, BSN, CNOR[b], Debra Denny, RN, MHA[a],
Melanie Stoia, RN, BSN[a]

**KEYWORDS**

- Hybrid • Interventional radiology • Operating room
- Endovascular • Redesign • Competency

The benefits of hybrid operating suites that combine the technology and environments needed for open surgical repair and radiology-dependent, less invasive interventional work are well documented. At Baptist Cardiac and Vascular Institute, the utility, safety, and effectiveness of a hybrid interventional radiology (IR) suite continues to be demonstrated with optimal patient outcomes for endovascular aneurysm repair (EVAR) procedures. Redesign and upgrades to the room were done and include higher quality imaging, more efficient and safer equipment, and integrated diagnostic tools and monitors for improved accuracy. Operational and cost efficiency measures were also achieved by cross-training IR nurses and radiologic technologists (RTs) to perform functions of the operating room (OR) circulating nurse and scrub technician (ST), creating a team of highly competent "hybrid" staff. The expanding scope of interventional work to intricate cardiology, neuroradiology, oncology, and pulmonary applications in the hybrid interventional environment requires well-trained and highly competent staff that can perform in the most simple to complex combined interventional and open surgical procedures.

## REDESIGN OF A WELL-ESTABLISHED HYBRID IR SUITE PERFORMING ENDOVASCULAR PROCEDURES

The benefits of hybrid operating suites that combine the technology and environments needed for open surgical repair and radiology-dependent, less-invasive interventional work are well documented.[1-5] At Baptist Cardiac and Vascular Institute (BCVI), the

From the Baptist Cardiac and Vascular Institute, Miami Florida. Funding and technical support for this project were provided by the Baptist Cardiac and Vascular Institute and Baptist Health South Florida.

[a] Baptist Cardiac and Vascular Institute, Baptist Hospital of Miami, 8900 North Kendall Drive, Miami, FL 33176, USA

[b] Organizational Learning, Baptist Health South Florida, 8500 SW 177 Avenue Road, Miami, FL 33183, USA

* Corresponding author.
*E-mail address:* janek@baptisthealth.net

Perioperative Nursing Clinics 5 (2010) 215–227
doi:10.1016/j.cpen.2010.02.002
1556-7931/10/$ – see front matter © 2010 Elsevier Inc. All rights reserved.

development of a hybrid endovascular suite began in 1993. An existing, albeit, state-of-the-art angiography room was modified to meet all patient care, workflow, infection control, and regulatory requirements to perform combined surgical and interventional procedures (**Fig. 1**). Since then, many facilities have reported adoption of the hybrid concept, primarily in the OR environment. Technology native to radiology and cardiac catheterization labs is installed in a traditional OR, allowing the surgeon and the interventional physician to perform combined services in one session without moving the patient.

The decision to create a hybrid IR suite rather than a hybrid OR suite at BCVI was made by a collaborative group of vascular surgery and IR representatives. Even though endovascular grafts as a method of treatment for aneurysms was in its infancy, the promise of combined surgical and interventional procedures was clear. The goal was to create an environment that would fully support imaging and interventional capabilities, surgery, anesthesia, and provide optimal patient care for a variety of procedures. The team completed a comprehensive assessment of the existing imaging equipment in the ORs and the angiography-interventional suite. Also reviewed were the key resource requirements for endograft procedures. It was agreed that endograft procedures are heavily dependent on high-quality imaging and interventional skills and tools, but that typical interventional suites lack several features required for optimal surgical patient care. Endograft deployment requires surgical access because of the size of the grafts but is guided entirely by imaging. Imaging equipment in the OR was primarily used as an adjunct to surgical procedures and produced limited, low-quality views. Placement of new, high-quality imaging equipment in the OR was not possible because of low ceilings and existing design limitations. Also considered was the restricted scope of applicable service the high-end equipment would have in the OR, resulting in a lack of return on the investment. A

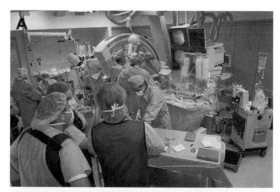

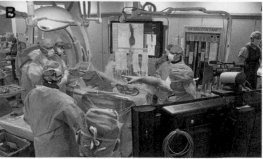

**Fig. 1.** Angiography room before (*A*) and after (*B*) renovation.

multidisciplinary team of physicians and staff from IR, vascular surgery, anesthesia, critical care, infection control, surgical services, nursing, quality assurance, and risk management was developed to plan and implement a hybrid IR suite.

The original hybrid suite that was developed included all of the critical elements to support combined surgical and interventional procedures. The suite measured 600 sq ft,[6] suspended ceiling surgical lights were installed, a variety of tables and trays were brought in, and storage space was designed for immediate access to angiographic catheters, wires, and equipment. Room modifications were made to ensure 20 to 25 air exchanges per hour, at least 20% with fresh air,[7–9] positive air pressure in the procedure room relative to surrounding corridors,[7–9] temperature of 65° to 75°F (18°–24°C),[7–9] humidity of 50% to 55%,[7–9] washable ceilings to avoid contamination with bacteria-harboring dust particles,[10] seamless floors with integral wall bases to avoid areas that could harbor bacteria,[10] disinfection preparation of the procedure suite,[7,11,12] pre-procedural scrub area for personnel, and adequate traffic control and barriers to access during combined procedures.[7,9,11,12] The imaging equipment included an Integris V-3000 (Philips, Best, The Netherlands) that was washable and disinfected between cases with a bleach solution. Extensive cross-training was conducted to develop core competencies; interventional technical and nursing staff were trained on surgical technique, surgical scrub and traffic flow; and surgical staff were trained in radiation protection and working in a fluoroscopic environment. Cross-training was done on endovascular procedure technique and emergency conversion to open surgical procedures. All endovascular procedures included an OR team, including a vascular surgeon, surgical assistant, and scrub nurse; one anesthesiologist; and an IR team including the interventional radiologist, fellow, RT, IR nurse, and one assistant. Although the environment was deemed suitable for open surgery when renovations were completed, initial plans were to transport the patient to the OR if conversion was necessary since it could be accomplished in less than 10 minutes.

## RESULTS

Sixteen years later, the utility, safety, and effectiveness of the hybrid IR continues to be demonstrated through optimal patient outcomes, a highly collaborative work team and a high room-use rate with combined and solely interventional procedures routinely performed in the room. Over 1000 aortic and thoracic aneurysm and endovascular stent repairs have been done. Adverse events requiring conversion to open surgical repair have been rare and have not required moving the patient to the OR since all equipment and supplies are immediately available and the OR team was present. To date, no untoward effects from open surgical repair in the interventional suite have been reported. The average annual risk-adjusted mortality rate for uncomplicated patients at less than 1% supports the safety and efficacy of endovascular procedures in a hybrid IR environment.

## HYBRID IR REDESIGN

As interventional services evolved, advancements in technology and equipment kept pace. In 2007, the need for hybrid IR room upgrades was evident with the availability of higher quality, more efficient, and safer imaging equipment on the market. Improvements in technology include integration of diagnostic tools and imaging such as cone beam CT, intravascular ultrasound, 3D angiographic road mapping, and picture archiving and communication systems that provide immediate visualization and guidance for better clinical decision-making, accuracy, and patient outcomes. These features were added to the hybrid room as they became available from 2001 to 2007. Significant upgrades were still needed, however, and facility plans were developed. Upgrades to the room include installation of a Philips Allura FD20 with Flat Detector imager with a ceiling suspended C-arm for faster, more flexible rotational scans of complex vasculature images, a free-floating pivot table for ideal positioning of patients up to 550 lbs, and pulse fluoroscopy for reduced radiation doses to patients. The new imager also features technology that filters out "soft" radiation and minimizes scatter for a safer work environment for staff. Renovations also included new ceiling beams to support an easy to move boom to house oxygen and anesthesia lines, light-emitting diode surgical lighting, swing-arm radiation shielding, and a state-of-the-art Philips FlexVision XL LCD full color monitor. This 56 in, high-definition, flat-panel monitor allows up to eight images from multiple sources to be displayed simultaneously for superior quality images and information display to guide interventions. The team now appreciates a more open workspace with a majority of the equipment off the floor and out of the way.

## COST-EFFECTIVENESS

Though renovations produced a more efficient, safer environment, the high cost of endovascular procedures remained a concern. Review of operating expenses showed an opportunity to reduce expenses in both supply and labor resource use. Stent graft pieces alone range anywhere from $4,000 to $24,000 each, and highly sophisticated catheters and wires can cost several thousand dollars. We completed a focused review of supplies and worked collaboratively with physicians to standardize product when possible. A reduction in the number of staffing hours per procedure, however, proved to be our greatest opportunity for cost-reduction. Since the literature supports that staff members can effectively and efficiently participate in EVAR procedures with the proper training,[5] the decision was made to fully cross-train IR nurses and RTs to perform the functions of the OR circulating nurse and scrub technician, creating a team of well-qualified, highly skilled, hybrid registered nurses and RTs.

## PERIOPERATIVE CROSS-TRAINING OF IR STAFF
### Planning

The first step to begin the perioperative education program for IR staff was planning. Several meetings between the IR and OR directors, managers, and educators were necessary to determine the contributing roles of each specialty and the methods of teaching. Required surgical supplies and equipment typically provided by the OR for EVAR cases was also identified for purchase by the IR department. A timeline was established to determine the quantity and length of classroom sessions to be held, a date to begin, and a tentative date for completion of the program. A total of eleven registered nurses, RTs, and cardiovascular assistants needed to be cross-trained and attend the didactic portion of the program. A team of five, which included two nurses, two technologists, and one assistant, was selected to be the first team that would eventually work independently from the OR during EVAR procedures. Once competency was achieved by the first team, the second team of six would start training.

The next step was identifying the difference in roles and learning needs of the IR registered nurse to competently perform the role of the perioperative nurse and of the RT to perform the role of the ST. The two specialties vary in education and experience in regards to aseptic technique and OR standards of practice. Perioperative nurses attend formal educational classes with a curriculum developed by the Association of Perioperative Registered Nurses (AORN) to learn perioperative standards and recommended practices before working in the OR. Following a 10 to 12 week program, the novice OR nurse generally completes a competency-based orientation that extends 3 to 6 months, depending on the size of the OR and its varied specialties. A minimum of 1 year experience is expected before being considered a competent perioperative nurse. IR registered nurses usually have intensive care or emergency services experience with comprehensive education in critical care. A competency-based orientation ordinarily extends 3 months to learn the various procedures and requirements of working in a fluoroscopic environment.

Surgical technologists (STs) attend a 12-month surgical technology program from an accredited school, a course that includes a clinical externship. ST are taught

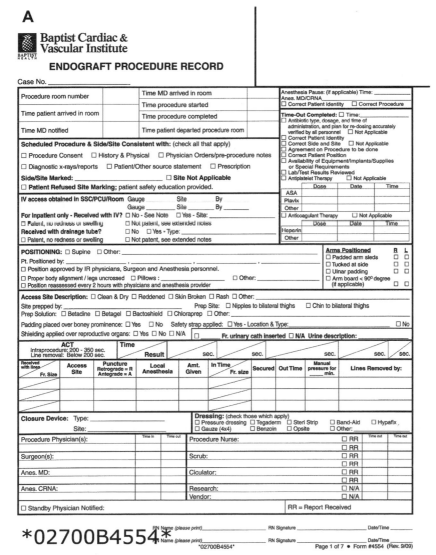

**Fig. 2.** Comprehensive procedure record. (*Courtesy of* the Baptist Cardiac and Vascular Institute; with permission.)

**B**

**Baptist Cardiac & Vascular Institute**
BAPTIST HEALTH

## ENDOGRAPH PROCEDURE RECORD

**Specimens:**

☐ Type: _____    ☐ Disposition: _____

☐ Culture # _____    ☐ Frozen # _____    **Wound Class:**

☐ Permanent # _____    ☐ Other # _____    ☐ 1 Clean          ☐ 3 Contaminated

☐ See Supplemental    ☐ See Anesthesia Record          ☐ 2 Clean - contaminated    ☐ 4 Dirty

| Medication Record | | | | | | | | | | Confirm Patient's I.D. | | ☐ Procedure Room | | ☐ PCU | | | | | | | | |

| Effect<br>S = successful<br>U = unsuccessful | Quality of<br>Effort (QOE)<br>0 = Apenic<br>1 = Labored or limited<br>2 = Normal | Level of Consciousness<br>(LOC)<br>1 = Unresponsive<br>2 = Responds to painful stimuli<br>3 = Responds to physical stimuli<br>4 = Responds to verbal stimuli<br>5 = Alert/Awake | Distal pulses<br>✓ = No change<br>from<br>pre-procedure | Access Site<br>✓ = No bleeding,<br>no hematoma<br>* = Change -<br>see Nurse's<br>Notes | ECG<br>✓ = No change<br>from<br>pre-procedure<br>* = Changes -<br>see Nurse's Notes | Pain Intensity Scale<br>0 = None    6 = Severe<br>2 = Mild    8 = Very Severe<br>4 = Moderate    10 = Worst possible |

| Time | Medication | Dose | Route | Initials | Witness | Time | Effect | RN Initials | Time | HR | ECG | BP Cuff | A-line BP | Resp. R | QOE | O2 Sat | Oxygen | ETCO2 | Access Site | Distal Pulse | Pain Score | LOC |
|------|-----------|------|-------|----------|---------|------|--------|-------------|------|----|----|---------|-----------|---------|-----|--------|--------|-------|-------------|--------------|------------|-----|
| | | | | | | | | | | | | | | | | | | | | | | |
| | | | | | | | | | | | | | | | | | | | | | | |
| | | | | | | | | | | | | | | | | | | | | | | |
| | | | | | | | | | | | | | | | | | | | | | | |
| | | | | | | | | | | | | | | | | | | | | | | |
| | | | | | | | | | | | | | | | | | | | | | | |
| | | | | | | | | | | | | | | | | | | | | | | |
| | | | | | | | | | | | | | | | | | | | | | | |
| | | | | | | | | | | | | | | | | | | | | | | |
| | | | | | | | | | | | | | | | | | | | | | | |
| | | | | | | | | | | | | | | | | | | | | | | |
| | | | | | | | | | | | | | | | | | | | | | | |

**Pulse Criteria**
2 = strong palpable    2D = strong doppler    0 = none
1 = weak palpable    1D = weak doppler

**Dialysis Access**
B: Bruit
T: Thrill

| | Femoral | | Dorsalis pedis | | Posterior tibial | | Radial | | Dialysis Access | | Labs/Tests | Done @ | Results | Reviewed by RN Initials |
|---|---------|---|----------------|---|------------------|---|--------|---|-----------------|---|-----------|--------|---------|-------------------------|
| PRE | L | R | L | R | L | R | L | R | L | R | | | | |
| POST | L | R | L | R | L | R | L | R | L | R | | | | |

(P U L S E S)

RN Name *(please print)* _____    RN Signature _____    Date _____ Time _____

RN Name *(please print)* _____    RN Signature _____    Date _____ Time _____

## *02700B4554*

*02700B4554*

Page 2 of 7 • Form #4554  (Rev. 9/09)

**Fig. 2.** (*continued*)

proper scrubbing, gowning, gloving, instrumentation, sterilization, and aseptic practices, as well as the many types of surgical procedures they will encounter while working as an ST. RT's attend a 2 or 4 year RT program from an accredited school to perform diagnostic imaging examinations and administer radiation therapy treatments. They are educated in anatomy, patient positioning, examination techniques, equipment protocols, radiation safety, radiation protection, and basic patient care. Programs do not generally include interventional or surgical procedure education. RTs often subspecialize after graduation and complete 3 to 6 month competency-based orientations, depending on the specialty.

The last step of the planning phase included identifying the differences between the interventional environment versus the OR environment that would need to be

**C**

**Baptist Cardiac &
Vascular Institute**
BAPTIST HEALTH

**ENDOGRAFT PROCEDURE RECORD**

| NURSING PLAN OF CARE |
|---|

**Potential for injury, infection and alteration in skin integrity**

| Goal | Outcome |
|---|---|
| _____ Positions patient to maintain respiration and circulation. | _____ Patient is free from injury related to the nursing process. |
| _____ Applies principles of aseptic technique. | _____ Patient had no or minimal exposure to exogenous wound contamination. |
| _____ Uses CDC guidelines for defining surgical site. | _____ Patient skin integrity is maintained. |

☐ See Perioperative Fluid Record  **INTAKE**  **OUTPUT**

| Time | Site | IV Solution | Rate | Amt. hung / Amt. received | Amt. Infused | Stop Time | Time | Urine | Other |
|---|---|---|---|---|---|---|---|---|---|
|  |  |  |  |  |  |  |  |  |  |
|  |  |  |  |  |  |  |  |  |  |
|  |  |  |  |  |  |  |  |  |  |

| Time | Route | Medication / Irrigation to Field | Dosage | | **Thermal Unit** |
|---|---|---|---|---|---|
|  |  |  |  |  | ☐ Unit #: _____ |
|  |  |  |  |  | Temperature setting: _____ |
|  |  |  |  |  | ☐ Upper body   ☐ Under body |
|  |  |  |  |  | Barrier between patient and thermal blanket. ☐ YES  ☐ NO |

| Counts | Correct | Incorrect | N/A | # | **Electrocautery:** |
|---|---|---|---|---|---|
| Sponge |  |  |  |  | Unit #: _____ |
| Sharps |  |  |  |  | Settings Coag: _____  Cut: _____ |
| Instruments |  |  |  |  | Location of Grounding Pad: _____ |
| Other |  |  |  |  | ☐ Skin Intergrity Assessment Completed |

☐ Surgeon notified of count results    *RT performing count:* _____

☐ Pre-procedure  ☐ Post-procedure

☐ Actions taken for incorrect count  ☐ N/A   *RN performing count:* _____

Comments: _____

X-Ray taken ☐ Yes ☐ No      Waived instrument count: ☐ Yes ☐ No

Read by: _____       ☐ Reason: _____

Findings: ☐ Negative (-) ☐ Positive (+)

_____

**Procedure completed:** _____

_____

| Fluoro: | | **CONTRAST USED** | | | | | | |
|---|---|---|---|---|---|---|---|---|
| Time: _____ minutes | | Type and Dose | **VIAL SIZE in ml** | | | | | TOTALS |
| | | | 15 | 20 | 50 | 100 | 150 | |
| **Dose:** | Injector | | | | | | | |
| Rm. 7 _____ Gycm² | 1. | | | | | | | ml |
| Rm. 2 & 5 _____ mGycm² | 2. | | | | | | | ml |
| **Maximum Dose:** | Table | | | | | | | |
| **2,110 Gycm² or 2,110,000 mGycm²=1500 rads for IVR patients. | 1. | | | | | | | ml |
| **1,050 Gycm² or 1,050,000 mGycm²=1500 rads for CVL patients. | 2. | | | | | | | ml |

RN Name *(please print)* _____   RN Signature _____   Date _____ Time _____

RN Name *(please print)* _____   RN Signature _____   Date _____ Time _____

**\*02700B4554\***

\*02700B4554\*                Page 3 of 7 ● Form #4554  (Rev. 9/09)

**Fig. 2.** (*continued*)

addressed in the cross-training. IR staff would need to assume full responsibility for implementing and maintaining all OR controls and standards regarding traffic patterns,[13] environmental cleaning,[14] and strict surgical attire guidelines during open surgical procedures.[15] These standards were taught during the initial hybrid IR program training in 1993 and are currently being followed but with the OR teams lead. It was agreed that re-education of the expectations and principles would be necessary for complete understanding, reinforcement, and strict compliance to the AORN standards.

### Implementation

Classroom training was conducted for the 11 IR staff and included comprehensive education of the perioperative standards and recommended practices during EVAR

**D**

**Baptist Cardiac & Vascular Institute**
BAPTIST HEALTH

**ENDOGRAFT PROCEDURE RECORD**

| DATE | TIME | NURSE'S NOTES | NURSE'S INITIALS |
|------|------|---------------|------------------|
|      |      |               |                  |
|      |      |               |                  |
|      |      |               |                  |
|      |      |               |                  |
|      |      |               |                  |
|      |      |               |                  |
|      |      |               |                  |
|      |      |               |                  |
|      |      |               |                  |
|      |      |               |                  |
|      |      |               |                  |
|      |      |               |                  |
|      |      |               |                  |
|      |      |               |                  |
|      |      |               |                  |
|      |      |               |                  |
|      |      |               |                  |
|      |      |               |                  |
|      |      |               |                  |
|      |      |               |                  |
|      |      |               |                  |
|      |      |               |                  |
|      |      |               |                  |
|      |      |               |                  |
|      |      |               |                  |
|      |      |               |                  |
|      |      |               |                  |
|      |      |               |                  |
|      |      |               |                  |
|      |      |               |                  |
|      |      |               |                  |
|      |      |               |                  |

RN Name *(please print)*_____   RN Signature _____   Date _____ Time _____

RN Name *(please print)*_____   RN Signature _____   Date _____ Time _____

**\*02700B4554\***

\*02700B4554\*                     Page 4 of 7  •  Form #4554  (Rev. 9/09)

**Fig. 2.** (*continued*)

procedures: appropriate procedural attire; asepsis, including aseptic principles and sterile techniques; environmental cleaning; sterilization and decontamination, including the use of process indicators; wound classification; and name and function of the cardiovascular instruments used during the endovascular procedure. Also covered were proper handling and passing of instruments; positioning with a review of common positioning injuries; proper technique for skin preparation and the different types of antimicrobial products used for patients to prevent infection; scrubbing, gowning, and gloving; protocols for instrument, sponge, and sharp counts before, during, and after the procedure; patient and personnel safety factors during use of electrosurgery; names and uses for suture; and review of the surgeons' preference cards.

E

**Baptist Cardiac & Vascular Institute**
BAPTIST HEALTH

**ENDOGRAFT PROCEDURE RECORD**

**DEVICE TRACKING**
(Place implant sticker in correspoding box)

| Implant(s): | Implant(s): | Implant(s): |
|---|---|---|
| | | |
| Site _____ | Site _____ | Site _____ |
| Time _____ | Time _____ | Time _____ |

| Implant(s): | Balloon(s): | Balloon(s): |
|---|---|---|
| | Label | Label |
| | Site _____ | Site _____ |
| | Time _____ | Time _____ |
| | Label | Label |
| Site _____ | Site _____ | Site _____ |
| Time _____ | Time _____ | Time _____ |

RN Name *(please print)* _____   RN Signature _____   Date _____ Time _____
RN Name *(please print)* _____   RN Signature _____   Date _____ Time _____

**\*02700B4554\***   *02700B4554*   Page 6 of 7 • Form #4554  (Rev. 9/09)

**Fig. 2.** (*continued*)

Re-education on converting the traffic flow in the IR suite to the three designated zones (the unrestricted, semirestricted, and restricted areas) to meet open surgery standards was done. The BCVI IR suites are surrounded by an unrestricted outside corridor for patient access to procedure rooms. Conversion to a semirestricted area is achieved by closing the double doors at each end of the corridor and posting signs restricting access to IR personnel only. Non-IR personnel are prevented from entering this area during EVAR procedures.

## Teaching Methodology

The teaching strategies used included didactic classes with PowerPoint presentations followed by class discussions, demonstration and return demonstration, and a one-

**F**

**Baptist Cardiac & Vascular Institute**
BAPTIST HEALTH

### ENDOGRAFT PROCEDURE RECORD

| Post Procedure Nursing Plan of Care | | |
|---|---|---|
| **Nursing Diagnosis: Impaired gas exchange/pain/knowledge of deficit** | | |
| **Goal** | Optimal gas exchange, physical and emotional and understanding of post-procedure teaching | **Recovery/Discharge Outcomes** |
| _____ | Respiratory rate, depth, oxygen saturation, vital signs, and level of consciousness assessed. | _____ Patient maintained optimal neurologic and cardiopulmonary functions. |
| _____ | Safety measures initiated as necessary. | _____ Patient is awake and cognizant of surroundings. |
| _____ | Comfort measures provided. | _____ Patient emerged from sedation without complication. |
| _____ | Post-procedure/discharge teaching done. | _____ None or minimal discomfort. |
| | | _____ Patient/family/SO demonstrates understanding of post-procedure teaching. |

| Post Anesthesia Recovery Score (PARS)   ☐ See Post Anesthesia Care Unit Record form # 4510 | | Discharge |
|---|---|---|
| **Activity** | 0 = Unable to lift head or move extremities. | |
| | 1 = Moves two extremities voluntarily or on command and can lift head. | |
| | 2 = Able to move four extremities voluntarily or on command. Can lift head. | |
| **Respiration** | 0 = Apneic. Condition necessitates ventilator or assisted respiration. | |
| | 1 = Labored or limited respirations. May have mechanical airway. | |
| | 2 = Can take a deep breath and cough well. Has normal respiratory rate and depth. | |
| **Circulation** | 0 = Has abnormally high or low BP (greater than 50% presedation level). | |
| | 1 = BP 20% - 50% or presedation level. | |
| | 2 = Stable BP and pulse. (BP less than or equal to 20% of presedation level). | |
| **Neurologic** | 0 = Not responding or responding to painful stimuli. | |
| | 1 = Responds to verbal stimuli but drifts off to sleep easily. | |
| | 2 = Awake, alert, oriented to time, place and person. | |
| **O$_2$ Sat** | 0 = O$_2$ saturation less than 90% with O$_2$ supplement. | |
| | 1 = Needs O$_2$ inhalation to maintain O$_2$ saturation greater than 90% or less than 95%. | |
| | 2 = Able to maintain pre-procedure O$_2$ saturation on room air or greater than 95% on O$_2$. | |
| | **Total Recovery Score** | |

| IV discontinued at (time) _____ | ☐ No redness or swelling of site _____ | ☐ N/A |
|---|---|---|

RN Name *(print)* _____   RN Signature _____   Date _____ Time _____

RN Name *(print)* _____   RN Signature _____   Date _____ Time _____

☐ Patient discharged to inpatient room #: _____       ☐ Implant Card/Information provided to patient/designee (if applicable)
                                                        ☐ Implant Card/Information placed in chart (if applicable)

Belongings returned to patient/designee _____

Admitting Physician: _____   Time Notified _____ ☐ N/A

Post PCU Procedure Orders Verified by: _____ / _____ (Patients recovered in PCU only)
                                       PCU RN Name print        PCU RN Signature

Report given to: _____   Report given by: _____

Discharge RN: _____   Time of Discharge: _____

Patient Received by: _____ / _____ RN
                     Print                      Signature

## *02700B4554*

*02700B4554*       Page 7 of 7 ● Form #4554 (Rev. 9/09)

**Fig. 2.** (*continued*)

on-one demonstration of competencies using a competency skills checklist. The staff was given regular evaluation instruments throughout the program to test their knowledge.

Didactic classes were held for 6 weeks, followed by 9 weeks of classes in the procedure room. The majority of the learning took place while in the procedure room, practicing all the necessary skills and knowledge required to assist during EVAR procedures. Each staff member completed their competency skills and met all objectives. A 1-hour class was also held for the IR physicians that focused on surgical site infections and aseptic practices during IR procedures.

Initially, IR nurses and RTs felt out of their realm of comfort performing the functions of the perioperative nurse and ST. With close preceptor oversight, support, and constructive feedback the staff were able to develop the skills, competence, and confidence to assist the interventional physicians and the vascular surgeons in combined interventional and open surgical EVAR cases. The performance expectations of each role have become normal standard of care for all patients and procedures, no matter how simple or complex. OR registered nurses and scrub technicians labor expenses have decreased by an average of 7 hours per procedure.

### Challenges

As with any new venture, there are always challenges. The main challenges encountered included:

1. Finding time for classes and training was a challenge because staff needed to be available to work in scheduled procedures and to keep the department fully operational. The classes were held every Wednesday morning from 7:00 AM to 8:30 AM and a delayed start time for the department was approved.
2. OR personnel were assigned as preceptors to work with individual IR staff during the EVAR procedures. Pre-procedure sessions were planned so the teams could meet before to discuss issues and concerns. Because of different work schedules and competing priorities, the two teams were not able to meet before cross-training and preceptor sessions.
3. The physical layout of the hybrid IR room is long and narrow with stationary radiology equipment, creating the challenge of keeping traffic away from the sterile field.

### OTHER PROCESS CHANGES

Once the program began, the need to merge required IR and OR data fields onto one tool for documentation was apparent. All elements of patient assessment, intervention, evaluation, procedures performed, "time-out" completion, device tracking, radiation exposure, and so forth had to be incorporated to a single, user-friendly procedure record to ensure compliance. **Fig. 2** illustrates the comprehensive procedure record developed by nursing staff that satisfies all regulatory and medical-legal standards of documentation. Although currently completed in hardcopy format, plans to convert to a fully integrated electronic medical record are in process.

### SUMMARY

Hybrid IR suites and cross-trained, hybrid staff for combined interventional and surgical procedures provide a safe and cost effective approach to health care. Although there are challenges to creating and maintaining a safe environment for open surgical procedures outside of the OR, effective measures can be taken. With careful planning, focused education, and flexible, highly collaborative work teams, staff can assume roles and responsibilities within their scope of practice that maximize competency and operational efficiencies.

### FUTURE CONSIDERATIONS AND CONCLUSIONS

The benefits and optimal resource use of the hybrid angiographic environment for a diverse group of procedures is more evident as new techniques are introduced and clearly supports the vision of the early pioneers of the hybrid environment such as the BCVI team. Advancements in technology as well as supplies that are more sophisticated, implants, medications, embolic and chemotherapeutic agents, and so forth, have expanded the scope of interventional work to intricate cardiology, neuroradiology, oncology, and pulmonary applications that could only be accomplished by more invasive, open surgery in the past.

At BCVI, procedures such as percutaneous structural heart procedures (closure of patent foramen ovale, atrial septal defects, atrial appendage, and mitral valve repair) are routinely done in the cardiac catheterization laboratory. These less-invasive, highly successful procedures require standby cardiothoracic surgical teams in the event that life-threatening complications occur. Though rare, complications such as cardiac tamponade or perforation can occur and require immediate intervention with no time to transfer to an OR suite. These and other routine but higher risk procedures further emphasize the need to have highly skilled, hybrid teams throughout all of the interventional service areas. Cross-training of the catheterization laboratory RNs and RTs to assist with initial open chest surgical intervention is in process.

Maintaining tight controls and out-of-the-box thinking by vascular surgeons, interventional radiologists, interventional cardiologists, and cardiothoracic surgeons will continue to expand future applications in the hybrid interventional suite. It is imperative that staff be prepared, well-trained, and competent to meet the demands of performing in the most simple to complex combined interventional and open surgical procedures.

## REFERENCES

1. Katzen BT, Becker GJ, Mascioli CA, et al. Creation of a modified angiography (endovascular) suite for transluminal endograft placement and combined interventional-surgical procedures. J Vasc Interv Radiol 1996;7:161–7.
2. Cantrell S. Outfitting the inner sanctum: trends in surgical suites. Healthcare Purchasing News. February 2009. p. 13–5.
3. Bell KE, Lopez AC. Hybrid repair of thoracoabdominal aneurysms: a combined endovascular and open approach. J Vasc Nurs 2008;26(4):101–8.
4. Zhao DH, Leacche M, Balaguer JM, et al. Routine intraoperative completion angiography after coronary artery bypass grafting and 1-stop hybrid revascularization: results from a fully integrated hybrid catheterization laboratory/operating room. J Am Coll Cardiol 2009;53(3):232–41.
5. Tinkham MR. The endovascular approach to abdominal aortic aneurysm repair. AORN 2009;89(2):289–306.
6. Altemeier WA, Burke JF, Clowes GH Jr, et al. Hospital design requirements for safe surgery. In: Altemeier WA, Burke JF, Pruitt BA Jr, et al, editors. Manual on control of infection in surgical patients (American College of Surgeons Committee on control of surgical infections of the committee on pre- and postoperative care). 2nd edition. Philadelphia: Lippincott; 1984. p. 269–70.
7. Altemeier WA, Burke JF, Clowes GH Jr, et al. Preparation and maintenance of a safe operating room environment. In: Altemeier WA, Burke JF, Pruitt BA Jr, et al, editors. Manual on control of infection in surgical patients (American College of Surgeons Committee on control of surgical infections of the committee on pre- and postoperative care). 2nd edition. Philadelphia: Lippincott; 1984. p. 111–20.
8. Nichols RL. The operating room. In: Bennett JV, Brachman PS, Sanford JP, editors. Hospital infections. 3rd edition. Boston (MA): Little, Brown; 1992. p. 461–7.
9. Soule BM. The APIC curriculum for infection control practice. Dubuque: Kendall Hunt Publishing Company; 1983. p. 850–1.

10. The Florida Legislature, Florida Statutes on Hospital Licensure, XXIX Public Health, Chapter 395.005 FS. Law implemented 395.001, 395.005 FS. History – New 1-1-77. Formerly 10D-28-82, Amended 9-3-92; 59A-3.082; 18:81–82.
11. Rutala WA. APIC guideline for selection and use of disinfectants. AJIC 1990;18:100–77.
12. Lange K. Recommended practices for sanitation in the surgical practice setting. AORN 1975;21:251–4.
13. Conner R. Recommended practices for traffic patterns in the perioperative practice setting. In: Perioperative standards and recommended practices. Denver: AORN Inc; 2009. p. 327.
14. Conner R. Recommended practices for surgical attire. In: Perioperative standards and recommended practices. Denver: AORN Inc; 2009. p. 299–301.
15. Conner R. Recommended practices for environmental cleaning in the preoperative setting. In: Perioperative standards and recommended practices. Denver: AORN Inc; 2009. p. 439.

# Uterine Fibroid Embolization for Symptomatic Leiomyomas: Perioperative Care

Jaime Lee, MSN, ARNP

**KEYWORDS**

- Uterine fibroid • Uterine fibroid embolization • UFE
- Uterine artery embolization • UAE • Uterine leiomyoma

## UTERINE FIBROIDS

Uterine fibroids, also known as uterine myomas or leiomyomas, are benign tumors of the myometrium that are found in 70% to 80% of all women of reproductive age.[1] Although these statistics seem daunting, most women with uterine fibroids remain asymptomatic. According to Spies and Czeyda-Pommersheim,[1] only 20% to 30% of uterine fibroids cause morbidity. The symptoms most commonly caused by leiomyomas include menorrhagia (heavy menstrual bleeding) and anemia as well as bulk-related symptoms such as pain (pelvic, low back, flank, legs), pelvic pressure, abdominal bloating and increased girth, urinary symptoms (frequency, urgency, nocturia, incontinence, ureteral compression leading to hydronephrosis), and constipation.

The bleeding pattern most typical of leiomyomas includes severe menorrhagia with prolonged cycles, generally as a result of submucosal and intramural fibroids, which distort the endometrial lining of the uterus (**Fig. 1**).[2] The actual mechanism by which fibroids cause menorrhagia remains unknown but many theorize that they compress veins within the uterus, thereby resulting in dilation of the veins within the endometrium.[3] Along with this heavy, lengthy cycle, many women experience iron-deficiency anemia and frequently require iron supplementation via oral medications as well as iron infusions and even blood transfusions. Severe menorrhagia is not only a source of medical concern but is routinely a source of stress and embarrassment for the patient as passage of a large vaginal clot and flooding of blood make it nearly impossible to maintain a normal way of life during menstruation (some women need to

Interventional Radiology Department, Georgetown University Hospital, 3800 Reservoir Road NW, Suite GG012, Washington, DC 20007, USA
*E-mail address:* jbk4@gunet.georgetown.edu

Perioperative Nursing Clinics 5 (2010) 229–239
doi:10.1016/j.cpen.2010.02.009
1556-7931/10/$ – see front matter

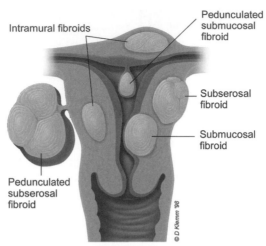

**Fig. 1.** Types of uterine fibroids. Fibroid classification is based on the position of the center of the fibroid in relationship to the uterus. Most fibroids are of mixed type. Intracavitary (not shown): fibroids completely inside the actual cavity of the uterus. These fibroids usually cause menorrhagia and severe cramping (depending on the size, they may be removed vaginally through a technique called hysteroscopic resection). Intramural: fibroids built into the wall of the uterus and expand inward. They usually cause uterine enlargement and thus bulk symptoms result. They also cause menorrrhagia as a result of distortion of the endometrium. These fibroids are common. Subserosal: fibroids found within the outside wall of the uterus that usually do not cause many symptoms unless they become large enough to expand outward and exert a mass effect on other neighboring organs. They typically do not affect menstruation, but can cause discomfort (pain and pressure). Submucosal: fibroids partially intruding into the endometrial cavity that are partially built within the wall of the uterus. They can cause menorrhagia as well as spotting/interperiod bleeding. Pedunculated: fibroids that can be submucosal and serosal but that have now grown a stalk (peduncle). These fibroids typically cause pressure symptoms by compressing adjacent organs. Ones that are positioned anteriorly typically cause urinary symptoms and similarly, those that are posteriorly positioned, cause rectal pressure and constipation. (*Courtesy of* David Klemm/Dr James Spies and Georgetown University Hospital; with permission.)

change their sanitary protection as often as every 15 minutes because of saturation). Interperiod bleeding/spotting is not characteristic of uterine fibroids and thus should be investigated to rule out a gynecologic carcinoma or other endometrial disease.[1]

Bulk-related symptoms associated with uterine fibroids are seemingly mostly related to the location of the fibroids (see **Fig. 1**). As mentioned earlier, large submucosal and intramural leiomyomas are most likely to cause menorrhagia as they distort the endometrial lining of the uterus.[2] Pelvic pressure and bloating are usually related to adjacent organs being compressed as a result of a mass effect of fibroids. Distortion that is mainly anterior in nature will likely cause urinary symptoms, such as urgency, frequency, nocturia, and infrequently incontinence, and similarly distortion that is primarily posterior will likely cause rectal pressure and feelings of constipation. As fibroids enlarge it is not atypical to hear complaints of referred back, flank, and leg pain as well.

Because fibroids are hormonally driven, many primary care providers and gynecologists implement medical therapies for fibroid management as a first-line treatment. These therapies include the use of oral contraceptives pills (OCPs), gonadotropin-releasing hormone (GnRH) agonists, and oral and intramuscular progesterones.

Historically, if, after trying the modalities mentioned earlier, symptoms persist, surgical options, including myomectomy (removal of fibroids) and hysterectomy (removal of the uterus) have been used as mainstays for fibroid treatment. Symptomatic uterine fibroids account for 30% of all hysterectomies performed yearly in the United States.[4]

For women who wish to avoid major surgery, prolonged recovery time, and/or the permanent loss of reproductive ability, another option that is available. Since first reported by Goodwin and colleagues[5] in 1996, uterine fibroid embolization (UFE) has proved itself a safe and effective, formidable, minimally invasive alternative to surgery with longstanding results of symptomatic relief.[6–9] UFE allows for the injection of embolic material directly into the arterial supply of fibroids to occlude the feeding vessels and cause ischemia and tissue death (**Figs. 2** and **3**). As the fibroids become ischemic and nonviable, they shrink and the patient's baseline symptoms, once associated with fibroid presence, decrease or altogether resolve. This article discusses uterine fibroids and the typical perioperative course of UFE, including patient selection, preprocedural evaluation, periprocedural care, and postprocedure management.

## PATIENT SELECTION

Because many of the symptoms associated with uterine fibroids can also be caused by other disease processes (eg, endometriosis, endometrial polyps, endometrial cancer, ovarian cysts, adenomyosis) it is critical that all prospective patients undergo a thorough preprocedure evaluation to best determine their candidacy for UFE. The first step in working up the potential patient is to establish whether or not they have fibroids, via ultrasound (US) or magnetic resonance imaging (MRI) of the pelvis. Many physicians prefer MRI with and without intravenous contrast, as these images allow for greater anatomic detail of soft tissue and organs (identifying uterus, ovaries, and overall vascularity/viability of fibroids) and therefore describe not only the precise positioning of the fibroids within the uterus but also their size and vascularity.[10] MRI can also discern whether or not fibroids are being supplied by ovarian artery collaterals and therefore, if the decision is made to proceed with UFE, can assist in the overall planning of the procedure (the potential need to embolize ovarian arteries as well).

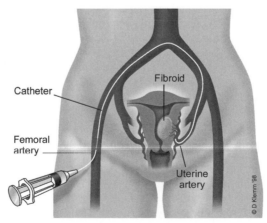

**Fig. 2.** Femoral access for uterine artery embolization. The catheter is within the uterine artery, which supplies most fibroids. (*Courtesy of* David Klemm/Dr James Spies and Georgetown University Hospital; with permission.)

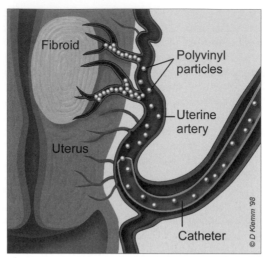

**Fig. 3.** Close-up of UFE. Embolic material traveling through the catheter within the uterine artery and occluding small feeder vessels to the fibroid. This process causes fibroid tissue ischemia and ultimately results in necrosis. (*Courtesy of* David Klemm/Dr James Spies and Georgetown University Hospital; with permission.)

Most women with uterine fibroids are asymptomatic and many have only trivial symptoms at most. Therefore, once the patient is found to have fibroids, the next question to ask is, do the symptoms truly warrant any intervention and if so, which intervention is most appropriate for this specific patient?

### Medical Therapy

Many medical practitioners ascribe to the theory of pursuing the least invasive technique first and then proceeding with more invasive maneuvers if necessary. As fibroids are largely estrogen driven, most algorithms for women presenting with menorrhagia, perhaps the most common symptom associated with uterine fibroids, include first trying medical therapies such as OCPs, GnRH agonists (to suppress ovarian activity and induce a hypoestrogenic state), and progesterones. In the absence of estrogen, myomas usually decrease in size and thus symptoms typically resolve. These effects are only temporary, as once the medications stop and there is a surge in estrogen, the fibroids typically rapidly grow back and symptoms recur. Another common complaint seen with uterine fibroids is that of dysmenorrhea (painful menstruation). Typically nonsteroidal antiinflammatory drugs (NSAIDs) are found to work well in reducing menstrual pain. Although there are many women for whom these transient therapies are effective, there are those who remain with symptoms, and those who cannot safely take these medications for other medical reasons (history of blood clots, allergies to NSAIDs, or gastric ulcers). In situations such as these other options must be explored.

### Myomectomy

As surgery has long been the mainstay treatment of uterine leiomyomas, there are 2 distinct options for women: myomectomy and hysterectomy. Appropriate candidacy for each option must be thoroughly explored with the patient. Myomectomy is a surgical option that allows for removal of the leiomyomas with uterine preservation. It is typically most widely used in young women with large uterine fibroids who wish to conceive in the future.[1] It is offered either abdominally or laparoscopically, as well as vaginally, depending on the uterine size as well as the location, size, and number of fibroids and depending on the skill of the surgeon. One of the main disadvantages of a myomectomy is the ineffectiveness of solving the underlying disease process. The incidence of subsequent surgery for leiomyomas following myomectomy is high, and has been reported at almost 5% per year.[11] Another study performed by Yoo and colleagues[12] suggests even higher recurrence rates. These investigators describe an incrementally steady increase in recurrence during the follow-up period and show 11.7% after 1 year, 36.1% after 3 years, 52.9% after 5 years, and 84.4% after 8 years. The transient nature of symptom relief secondary to this procedure leaves many women needing to undergo a second operation or seeking other therapeutic options.

## Hysterectomy

Although with a hysterectomy, the removal of the uterus eliminates all symptoms related to uterine fibroids as well as the potential for any future recurrence, it also removes any possibility for future childbearing.[13] This is a strong sticking point for many women of childbearing age. The most appropriate patient for a hysterectomy is typically one who either strongly desires this procedure to be performed, is not interested in potential childbearing, or one who is not a candidate for any other less invasive techniques for a variety of reasons. Some of these reasons include massively enlarged uteri, greater than 24 weeks' gestation, and women who have too many fibroids to count. Patients who have undergone multiple attempts at other treatment options and have failed to have symptom relief experience total symptom relief after undergoing a hysterectomy.

It is not uncommon that a hysterectomy is recommended to women based on their age as well as the presence of fibroids rather than the severity of the presenting symptoms. If a patient remains without symptoms then typically there is no justification for any intervention, let alone an invasive surgical one. There are some caveats to this rule, including hydronephrosis (dilatation of the collecting system as a result of ureteral obstruction), resulting from a mass effect of fibroids, as well as a uterine mass that may represent a gynecologic malignancy.[2] For these scenarios, a timely medical intervention is necessary to help preserve overall health and quality of life; this sometimes includes invasive surgery.

## UFE

Another option for treatment of uterine leiomyomas is UFE. Although it is still not yet considered part of the customary first line of options offered to patients by many physicians, Spies[2] found that most patients who present with symptomatic uterine fibroids are candidates for UFE. UFE is a minimally invasive procedure, performed under fluoroscopic guidance (real-time radiograph images). It allows for selective catheterization of the uterine arteries and injection of embolic material directly into the arterial supply of fibroids to occlude vessels and starve the fibroid of blood flow (see **Figs. 2** and **3**). This technique has been recognized as a safe and effective alternative to surgery by the American College of Obstetricians and Gynecologists[14] and recent data suggest that the therapeutic effect is durable and lasting.[7,8,15]

In general the size, location, and extent of fibroids determine a patient's appropriateness for the procedure. As overall success of UFE is measured by symptom relief, it is imperative to review the patient's baseline MRI and ensure that the most dominant fibroids in fact correlate with the prevailing symptoms for which the patient is presenting (see **Fig. 1**). If the patient is found to have negligible fibroids or symptoms unrelated to fibroids she must be referred elsewhere, as UFE would not be an appropriate intervention. Similarly, if on MRI the fibroids are found to be already avascular, then UFE would not provide any additional benefit and thus would not be appropriate.[2]

## PREPROCEDURAL EVALUATION

Besides reviewing a recent MRI (within 6 months) with the patient, a thorough assessment of the patient's gynecologic, medical, and surgical history by the radiologist is imperative for proper patient selection. Within the author's department at Georgetown University Hospital, it is typically required that the patient has undergone a comprehensive pelvic examination by a gynecologist within the past 6 months to a year. The author's department also requires that a Papanicolaou test has been performed within the past year and that it showed no abnormalities. For those patients who do present with a history of abnormal bleeding, especially for those who are postmenopausal, an endometrial biopsy is required within 6 months to exclude hyperplasia or endometrial malignancy.

A complete history of the present illness, including the patient's chief complaint, must be detailed. It is also important to ascertain information specific to bulk-related symptoms (eg, cramps, pelvic pain/pressure, bloating, urinary symptoms) in terms of severity as well as when in the cycle they tend to occur. Information regarding the patient's menstrual pattern is essential as well, specifically including data regarding frequency of occurrence, length of cycle, number of heavy days, number of pads/tampons used, and frequency of changing as a result of saturation. All of these data are used postprocedurally to make comparisons between symptoms before and after UFE and ultimately aid in determining overall patient satisfaction and success of treatment.

Once it has been determined that a patient is an appropriate candidate for this procedure, it is imperative to clearly discuss the risks, benefits, and alternatives to UFE with the patient so that she may make an educated decision on whether or not to proceed. Part of this determination is frequently based on the nature of the presumed recovery (eg, typical symptoms experienced, certain restrictions placed, time required off work). Presenting the patient with written documentation, outlining the common symptoms and scenarios associated with recovery, is beneficial and should be offered at the time of the initial consultation. This strategy allows the patient to study the material before the procedure and have a stronger understanding of her overall potential hospital and recovery course.

## PERIPROCEDURAL CARE

On the day of the procedure, the patient is admitted under the interventional radiology (IR) service and remains in the hospital for overnight observation after UFE. Once registered, the patient is brought to the holding area of the IR suite and asked to remove all clothing and change into a hospital gown. A complete history and focused physical examination are performed by a nurse practitioner or physician and informed consent is obtained. It does not matter whether or not the patient is menstruating as this procedure does not entail anything vaginally. If the patient is menstruating she must remove any tampons she is wearing and an absorbent pad is provided.

As this procedure is performed with conscious sedation via intravenous fentanyl citrate (Sublimaze) and midazolam (Versed), the patient should have fasted (remained with no food or fluid intake) since midnight the night before, except for taking necessary medications with a small sip of water. The specially trained IR nurse who provides sedation and analgesia should review the chart and verify that the patient understands the procedure and has no further questions.

## Preparation and Laboratory Examinations

Intravenous access should be obtained peripherally (18 or 20 gauge) and before starting any intravenous fluids (normal saline at a rate of 75 mL/h), 3 laboratory studies are required to be drawn and checked. A basic metabolic panel is checked to ensure that it is safe to proceed with conscious sedation (potassium levels <5.5 mEq/L) as well as to check renal function (creatinine) because intravenous contrast media will be used for fluoroscopic guidance. Because menorrhagia is the most common symptom associated with uterine fibroids, it is not uncommon for these patients to be anemic, and therefore a complete blood count needs to be performed before starting the procedure. If the patient is found to be severely anemic, a transfusion of packed red blood cells may be necessary (when applicable, consent is needed for this). Because pregnancy is an absolute contraindication for UFE, a urine pregnancy test (β-human chorionic gonadotropin) must be confirmed negative before any medications are given and before starting the procedure.

As this procedure requires the patient to receive either a unilateral or bilateral femoral arterial puncture, depending on the extent of the fibroids to be treated, the patient needs to remain on bedrest with legs extended for 2 to 6 hours after UFE depending on whether or not an arterial closure device was used. For this reason, a urinary catheter is sterilely placed into the patient's bladder and remains in place until the bedrest is complete. No preprocedural antibiotics are required.

## INTRAPROCEDURE

Once informed consent is obtained the patient is then taken into the IR suite where the procedure is performed. The patient is transferred onto the procedure table and prepared and draped in a sterile fashion. A baseline recording of all vital signs should be taken before the administration of any medication and should continue at a minimum every 5 minutes thereafter, until the conclusion of the procedure. This procedure is performed under conscious sedation, which is delivered by a trained and licensed health care professional, often a registered nurse. It is their primary responsibility during the case to monitor and attend to the patient, including monitoring the patient's vital signs as well as level of consciousness and level of comfort.

Intravenous diphenhydramine hydrochloride (Benadryl) provides a synergistic effect for sedating patients, via central nervous system depression, and can therefore allow for less overall dosing of narcotics and sedatives. The patient receives a 1-time dose of 50 mg of intravenous diphenhydramine at the start of the procedure. As it is an antihistamine, diphenhydramine also allows for coverage should the patient have an allergic response to the intra-arterial iodinated contrast that is injected during the procedure (something for which the registered nurse is monitoring). If the patient does have a known history of an allergy to contrast media, however, she is treated prophylactically with methylprednisolone (Medrol) 32 mg orally twice daily for 2 days before the scheduled procedure as well as receiving the dose of diphenhydramine mentioned earlier.

Intraoperatively, the patient receives 1 dose of ondansetron (Zofran) 4 mg for nausea prophylaxis as well as 2 doses of ketorolac (Toradol) 30 mg, 1 given at the start of the procedure and 1 at completion, to assist with pain management. These medications continue on a scheduled basis after the procedure for a period of 24 hours, at which point the patient should be able to tolerate oral intake, and is switched over to oral equivalents. A demand-only intravenous patient-controlled analgesia (PCA) pump, with morphine sulfate (less commonly fentanyl or hydromorphone) is also hung and primed at the conclusion of the procedure and is used throughout the patient's initial postprocedure course until she is able to tolerate oral narcotics.

## POSTPROCEDURAL MANAGEMENT
### Monitoring

Frequent monitoring of vital signs should continue every 15 minutes for the first hour after the last dose of medication was administered during the procedure. After the first hour, monitoring continues every 30 minutes for 1 hour, every hour for 4 hours and then per routine. At the immediate conclusion of the procedure, manual pressure is held over the groin puncture site until bleeding has stopped and sterile dressings are then placed over the sites. The groin puncture site should be checked and monitored during all vital sign checks, and if bleeding, oozing, or hematoma formation is noted, firm pressure should immediately be held directly over the artery, and should be maintained until the bleeding is controlled. If a pulsatile mass is observed at the groin puncture site, the IR team must be informed immediately, as this might indicate a pseudoaneurysm, which must be identified and treated quickly as it could rupture, requiring a surgical repair. Peripheral pulse checks (femoral, dorsalis pedis, and posterior tibialis) and skin temperature changes (cooling) should also be performed with all vital sign checks, as dissection of the artery as well as the potential for showering emboli are well-recognized complications of femoral artery catheterization. The pulse measurements should be checked against the patient's baseline and any changes should be communicated to the IR team.

While the patient is on bedrest, she should have bilateral pneumatic sequential stockings in place to decrease the potential for developing deep venous thrombosis (DVT). Many of these patients are already at an increased risk of thromboembolism because of their use of OCPs in an attempt to decrease menorrhagia and regulate their cycle. The pneumatic stockings may be removed once the patient is ambulatory, but thereafter they should remain on while the patient is in bed for any amount of time greater than 1 hour. If the patient has a well-documented history of DVT or pulmonary embolism she should be prophylactically treated with enoxaparin (Lovenox) immediately before the procedure and every 12 hours thereafter while in the hospital. Whether or not the patient needs to continue the regimen once discharged home depends on the treating/prescribing health care professional and should be taken on a case-by-case basis.

As intra-arterial iodinated contrast dye is used for fluoroscopic guidance during the procedure, the possibility of contrast-induced nephropathy remains a concern. A preprocedural chemistry panel is drawn and reviewed (specifically looking at creatinine levels) and all intake and output should be monitored. The author's department starts patients on an infusion of normal saline at 120 mL/h immediately after the procedure and this continues until the time of discharge, unless otherwise contraindicated, to ensure adequate hydration and renal clearance. Post-UFE oral and intravenous intake and urinary output must be measured and recorded routinely. The initial postprocedure period allows for ease in monitoring urinary output as the patient has a urinary catheter in place while she is on bedrest. After the hours of bedrest have passed, the catheter should be removed and a measuring device should be provided for the patient to use once she is ambulating to the bathroom and voiding independently.

### Pain and Nausea Management

Routine overnight care for patients' status after UFE should not only concentrate on monitoring the patient's stability but should also focus on providing pain relief and controlling symptoms of postembolization syndrome, including nausea/vomiting and significant fatigue as well as low-grade fever. These symptoms may be seen within the first few hours after the procedure and will likely continue to some degree throughout the first and second week of recovery. It is believed that these symptoms are a direct adverse effect of the fibroid/myometrial ischemia, although some believe the nausea to be related to the pain management regimen, as narcotics often cause nausea. Common management of these constitutional symptoms includes protocols that use a combination of intravenous narcotics (in the form of PCA) as well as scheduled doses of intravenous NSAIDs (Toradol) and antiemetics. As mentioned earlier, this regimen is started intraoperatively and is continued after the procedure until the patient is discharged home on oral equivalents.

### Care After Discharge

Typically on the morning following the procedure, the patient is discharged home. For this to occur, the patient must be tolerating a regular diet, must have pain that is at a tolerable level, and must be able to urinate spontaneously on her own after the catheter is removed. The patient is sent home with explicit written discharge instructions and contact information for the IR physicians, nurse practitioners, and office staff. She is given prescriptions for ibuprofen (Motrin) 800 mg every 6 hours for 4 days and then as needed, oxycodone 5 mg/acetaminophen 325 mg (Percocet) 1 to 2 tablets every 3 to 4 hours as needed for pain, and promethazine (Phenergan) 25 mg every 4 to 6 hours as needed for nausea.

As overall success of the procedure is entirely dependent on patient satisfaction, it is imperative that follow-ups with the patient occur to monitor this. Part of the

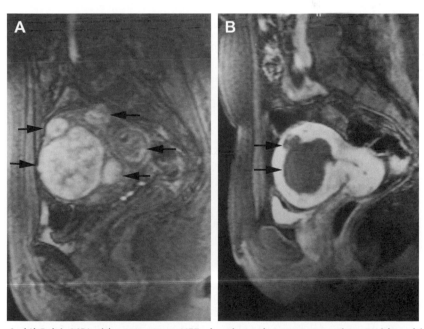

**Fig. 4.** (*A*) Pelvic MRI with contrast pre-UFE, showing enhancement consistent with multiple viable uterine fibroids (*arrows*). (*B*) Pelvic MRI with contrast 3 months after UFE shows no enhancement of the fibroids consistent with fibroid infarction (*arrows*). Only 2 of the fibroids are visible on this single image. Note the overall reduction in uterine size. (*Courtesy of* Dr James Spies.)

postprocedure management plan should entail contacting the patient on the day after discharge to screen for adequacy of pain and nausea control as well as to assess for any potential complications that may be developing, such as fibroid passage (necrotic tissue expelling out of vaginal canal), which is rare. A 1-week follow-up phone call should take place as well to ensure that recovery has been without incident and that the patient is stable and without any complaints. Many patients have light vaginal spotting or bleeding and may notice a persistent brownish vaginal discharge for several days or weeks. They also frequently experience some menstrual cycle irregularities, in terms of timing, but most return to a routine menstruation pattern within 3 to 4 months. Within 7 to 14 days, most patients are able to return to work and their other typical daily activities with no restrictions.

The standard in-office follow-up should occur 3 to 6 months after the procedure, once the patient has undergone a postprocedure MRI. At that visit all baseline symptoms and complaints should be compared with their current presentation and pre-UFE and post-UFE images should be studied and compared (**Fig. 4**).

## SUMMARY

Although several different therapeutic options exist for women with uterine leiomyomas, surgical options including myomectomy and hysterectomy have largely remained the standard approach. UFE provides a safe alternative to surgery and allows for uterine preservation with longstanding results and benefits. It has become a widely accepted treatment option for women with symptomatic fibroids and should therefore be discussed with all patients who could potentially be candidates.

## REFERENCES

1. Spies J, Czeyda-Pommersheim F. Uterine fibroid embolization. In: Mauro M, Murphy K, Thomson K, et al, editors. Image guided interventions. Philadelphia: Saunders Elsevier; 2008. p. 877–85.
2. Spies JS. Uterine fibroid embolization. In: Baum R, Pentecost M, editors. Abrams' angiography interventional radiology. Philadelphia: Lippincott Williams & Wilkins; 2006. p. 801–19.
3. Farrer-Brown G, Beilby JO, Tarbit MH. Venous changes in the endometrium of myomatous uteri. Obstet Gynecol 1971;38(5):743–51.
4. Myers ER, Barber MD, Gustilo-Ashby T, et al. Management of uterine leiomyomata: what do we really know? Obstet Gynecol 2002;100(1):8–17.
5. Goodwin SC, McLucas B, Lee M, et al. Uterine artery embolization for the treatment of uterine leiomyomata midterm results. J Vasc Interv Radiol 1999;10(9):1159–65.
6. Hutchins FL, Worthington-Kirsch R, Berkowitz RP. Selective uterine artery embolization as primary treatment for symptomatic leiomyomata uteri. J Am Assoc Gynecol Laparosc 1999;6(3):279–84.
7. Katsumori T, Kasahara T, Akazawa K. Long-term outcomes of uterine artery embolization using gelatin sponge particles alone for symptomatic fibroids. AJR Am J Roentgenol 2006;186(3):848–54.
8. Spies JB, Bruno J, Czeyda-Pommersheim F, et al. Long-term outcome of uterine artery embolization of leiomyomata. Obstet Gynecol 2005;106(5 Pt 1):933–9.
9. Pinto I, Chimeno P, Romo A, et al. Uterine fibroids: uterine artery embolization versus abdominal hysterectomy for treatment–a prospective, randomized, and controlled clinical trial. Radiology 2003;226(2):425–31.

10. Andrews RT, Spies JB, Sacks D, et al. Patient care and uterine artery embolization for leiomyomata. J Vasc Interv Radiol 2009;20(Suppl 7):S307–11.
11. Reed SD, Newton KM, Thompson LB, et al. The incidence of repeat uterine surgery following myomectomy. J Womens Health (Larchmt) 2006;15(9):1046–52.
12. Yoo EH, Lee PI, Huh CY, et al. Predictors of leiomyoma recurrence after laparoscopic myomectomy. J Minim Invasive Gynecol 2007;14(6):690–7.
13. Stewart EA. Uterine fibroids. Lancet 2001;357(9252):293–8.
14. Committee on Gynecologic Practice, American College of Obstetricians and Gynecologists. ACOG committee opinion. Uterine artery embolization. Obstet Gynecol 2004;103(2):403–4.
15. Goodwin SC, Spies JB, Worthington-Kirsch R, et al. Uterine artery embolization for treatment of leiomyomata: long-term outcomes from the FIBROID registry. Obstet Gynecol 2008;111(1):22–33.

# Vertebral Augmentation

Marion L. Growney, MSN, ACNP[a],*, Joshua A. Hirsch, MD[b,c]

**KEYWORDS**

• Vertebra • Augmentation • Osteoporosis • Fracture

Osteoporosis (porous bones) is a preventable condition in which bones become excessively weakened and prone to fracture. It is often called the silent disease because it does not have any symptoms until the patient suffers a fracture. Every year, more than 750,000 Americans sustain vertebral compression fractures.[1] Most of these fractures are attributed to osteoporosis, but a substantial amount are related to hematopoietic neoplasms, metastatic disease, or trauma. Osteoporotic vertebral fractures are often caused by routine activity such as stepping off a curb or opening a drawer. These types of fractures have an incidence of 25% in women more than 50 years of age. The National Osteoporosis Foundation reports that approximately 10 million Americans have the disease, with women accounting for nearly 8 million.[2] They estimate that 1 in 2 women will suffer an osteoporotic fracture in her lifetime.

Vertebral compression fractures can be associated with severe disabling pain. It is generally described by patients as a sudden onset of back pain often associated with little or no trauma. The pain can be constant, sharp, and typically centered over the spine.[3] Patients often report difficulty standing, walking, and performing activities of daily living. In many cases pain renders the patient bedridden. Before the advent of vertebral augmentation, the only available treatment was conservative management with bed rest, bracing, and narcotic pain management. Using this treatment method, many patients may have a slow, progressive improvement in their pain within 2 to 12 weeks. Prolonged immobilization is associated with muscular atrophy, accelerated bone loss, loss of cardiac function, and risk of developing pneumonia, pressure sores, gastrointestinal distress due to prolonged narcotic use, and deep vein thrombosis. The effects are considerable, even among a healthy patient population. Because most of these patients are of advanced age or oncology patients, the risks substantially increase.

Vertebral augmentation in the forms of vertebroplasty and kyphoplasty are minimally invasive techniques during which spinal needles are placed into the fractured vertebra. Under fluoroscopic or computed tomography (CT) guidance, polymethyl

[a] NeuroInterventional Radiology, Massachusetts General Hospital, MA, USA
[b] Departments of Interventional Radiology, NeuroInterventional Radiology/Endovascular Neurosurgery, Minimally Invasive Spine Surgery, Massachusetts General Hospital, MA, USA
[c] Harvard Medical School, Boston, MA, USA
* Corresponding author.
E-mail address: mgrowney@partners.org

Perioperative Nursing Clinics 5 (2010) 241–254
doi:10.1016/j.cpen.2010.02.007
1556-7931/10/$ – see front matter © 2010 Elsevier Inc. All rights reserved.

methacrylate (PMMA) cement is then placed into the vertebral body with the goal of relieving pain and reducing disability. These techniques offer a solution to a common medical issue causing significant morbidity and mortality among the most vulnerable patients.

Vertebroplasty was first performed in 1984 in France by Galibert and colleagues[4] who used the procedure to treat a symptomatic vertebral hemangioma. They discovered that the stabilization of the pathologic vertebral body with PMMA provided considerable pain relief. The procedure then found wider application in Europe for the treatment of pain related to myeloma and metastatic lesions in the vertebral bodies.[5,6] Experience with vertebroplasty in the United States began in 1993 at the University of Virginia.[7] At that time it was being used predominantly for the treatment of osteoporotic fractures, and its use for associated height restoration had not been evaluated (**Figs. 1–6** show vertebroplasty techniques).

In 2000, kyphoplasty was introduced as a proprietary product of Kyphon, Inc. (Sunnyvale, CA) Kyphoplasty has the additional goal of height restoration. It uses the insertion and inflation of a balloon immediately before cement placement. Kyphoplasty offers the possible advantage of greater height restoration and kyphosis correction, although it requires greater bone manipulation and increased operator time. The inflation of the balloon is believed to aid in restoring vertebral body height and to address issues with spinal alignment.[8] A large, multicenter trial was recently published showing a measurable improvement in pain following kyphoplasty (**Figs. 7–12**).[9]

Despite the limitations of traditional therapy, vertebroplasty, and kyphoplasty are typically reserved for patients who have failed conservative management because of the lack of randomized studies validating the efficacy of the procedure as a primary treatment. Currently, there are many case series on the effectiveness of vertebroplasty or kyphoplasty on pain relief with low complication rates.[3,10–18]

Sacroplasty is an emerging technology. Sacroplasty uses the techniques and materials of vertebral augmentation in sacral insufficiency fractures. However, there are few large studies that evaluate and compare the effectiveness of these procedures for all patients in terms of patient population and cause of compression fracture.[5] In a large retrospective published by Jha and colleagues[19] in 2009 it was shown that vertebroplasty, kyphoplasty, and sacroplasty afford pain relief for a preponderance of patients who have failed medical management apart from the underlying cause of the fracture. There was no difference in pain outcomes between the types of procedures.

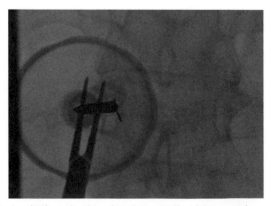

**Fig. 1.** Anteroposterior (AP) projection showing needle placement in vertebroplasty.

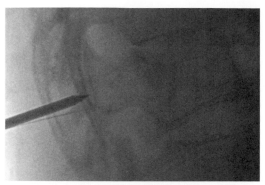

**Fig. 2.** Lateral projection showing needle placement during vertebroplasty.

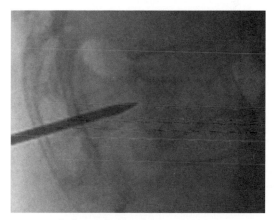

**Fig. 3.** Needle advancement during vertebroplasty.

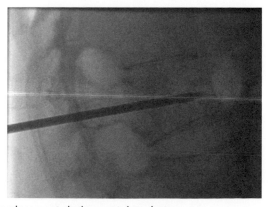

**Fig. 4.** Final needle placement during vertebroplasty.

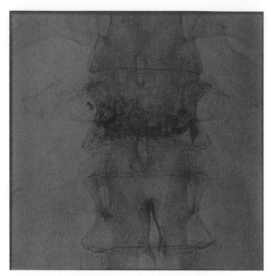

**Fig. 5.** AP image of cement placement after vertebroplasty.

Patient selection is a critical factor for achieving treatment success. A clinician plays a major role in correlating symptoms with imaging findings, and can exclude patients who are unlikely to benefit from vertebroplasty. Appropriate candidates have focal, midline back pain localized to the level of the fracture. Pain is worsened with bending, standing, or lifting, as the day progresses, and is decreased by lying flat in bed. Conventional radiography can be used to identify a new compression fracture, but radionuclide bone scans, magnetic resonance imaging (MRI) or CT is needed to determine whether the fracture is healed or not healed, especially in patients with multiple vertebral compressions. Indications for vertebral augmentation include painful vertebral compression fracture that has been refractory to medical therapy; painful vertebral hemangioma; painful metastatic lesion; painful fracture related to osteonecrosis, known as Kummel's disease; unstable vertebral compression fracture with movement of the wedge deformity; and reinforcement of vertebra before surgery. Healed fractures are generally not thought to benefit from vertebral augmentation.

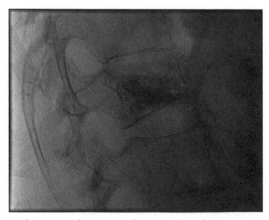

**Fig. 6.** Lateral image of cement placement after vertebroplasty.

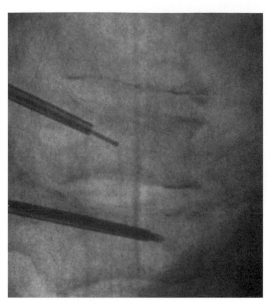

**Fig. 7.** Needle placement in 2-level kyphoplasty.

Back pain due to other problems such as disk disease and spinal stenosis must also be excluded. Advanced imaging also helps to distinguish osteoporotic fracture from metastasis or infection, and is necessary to ensure that vertebral augmentation can be performed safely.

Vertebral augmentation can be beneficial for oncology and osteoporotic patients suffering debilitating pain. Chemotherapy and radiation treatments commonly used to fight malignancy are also associated with resultant bone weakening, often leading to fracture. Many solid-tumor diseases are known to metastasize to the spine. Multiple myeloma is a cancer of the plasma cells. Myeloma is incurable but may have periods of remission induced by treatment. It has a multitude of symptoms including bone

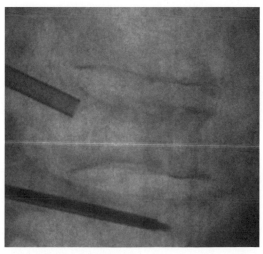

**Fig. 8.** Needle placement 2-level augmentation.

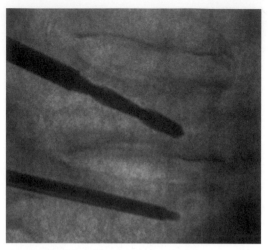

**Fig. 9.** Needle advancement in 2-level kyphoplasty.

pain, infection, renal failure, anemia, and neurologic symptoms. Myeloma pain typically involves the ribs and spine. Myeloma-related bone lesions are lytic in nature and may lead to pathologic fracture.

There are situations in which vertebral augmentation is not appropriate for the patient. The following are contraindications for vertebral augmentation procedures:

- Active infection
- Fractures that have lost more than 80% of height pose technical challenges and may not respond to treatment if displaced bone fragments are compressing the spinal cord or other neural structures
- Fractures caused by tumor infiltration may not be amenable to vertebral augmentation if there is cortical destruction and extensive epidural soft-tissue mass
- Patient must be able to lie prone for the duration of the procedure (most patients tolerate this position with conscious sedation)
- Presence of untreated coagulopathy
- Healed osteoporotic compression fractures

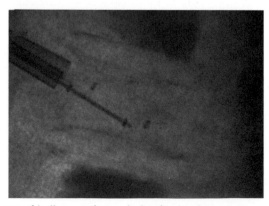

**Fig. 10.** Advancement of balloon catheter during kyphoplasty.

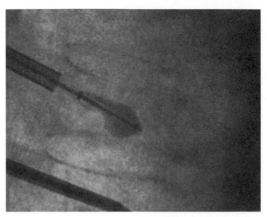

**Fig. 11.** Balloon inflation.

- Insufficient cardiopulmonary health needed to tolerate sedation or anesthesia
- Fracture-related compromise of the spinal canal sufficient to result in myelopathy or radiculopathy.

Vertebral augmentation is an image-guided minimally invasive procedure that is typically believed to be safe.[20] Risks are evident in every medical procedure. Vertebral augmentation has risks that are related to the needle placement, including bleeding, infection, and damage to any surrounding tissues, vessels, or bones. Risks related to the cement itself include cement leakage resulting in nerve irritation, damage or spinal canal compromise, and embolization into the lung. All image-guided procedures have the risk of radiation exposure. In more than 500 cases reported in 2009 by Jha and colleagues,[19] only 5 cases reported complications, and none required additional medical care or negatively affected patient well-being.

Vertebral augmentation may be performed in an outpatient setting that enables the patient to return home the same day. This outpatient option is attractive to many oncology patients who are already burdened with prolonged hospital stays. Many cases are preformed under procedural sedation that enables the patient to recover

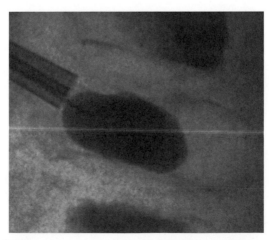

**Fig. 12.** Balloon inflation; note cement placement in adjacent levels.

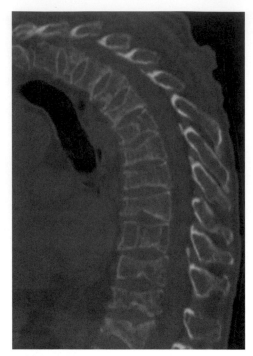

**Fig. 13.** Myeloma-related lytic lesions.

quickly and removes the added anesthesia risks. Postprocedure recovery involves approximately 3 hours of bed rest in a monitored recovery area. After the initial recovery period, patients are discharged to home with written instructions. It is recommended that they gradually increase their activity levels as tolerated in the days following the procedure. A small dressing is applied to the insertion site. The dressing may be removed after 24 hours and replaced with a dressing and antibiotic cream for 4 to 5 days until completely healed. Patients are seen in follow-up approximately 3 weeks after the procedure. At the time of follow-up, most patients report a substantial

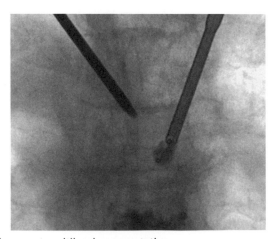

**Fig. 14.** Needle placement multilevel augmentation.

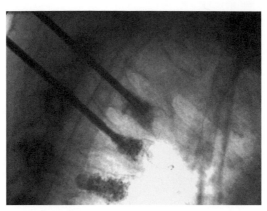

**Fig. 15.** Cement placement multilevel augmentation.

improvement in their fracture-related pain.[19] In that series, pain outcomes were not affected by the presence or absence of malignancy, the unilateral or bilateral needle placement approach, or the vertebral regions being treated per procedure (thoracic, lumbar, S1, or a combination of all 3). Comparable and large percentages of patients within each of these subcategories experienced pain improvement or resolution.[19]

## CASE STUDIES

A 70-year-old man presents to clinic with a history of sudden onset of back pain while lifting. He describes the pain as constant, centered over his spine, and debilitating. He

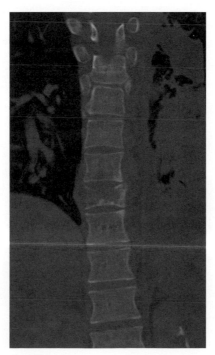

**Fig. 16.** Lytic lesion thoracic spine.

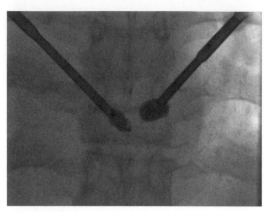

**Fig. 17.** Bipedicular kyphoplasty.

had initially presented to his primary care provider and was treated for muscle strain. He followed conservative management for several weeks without improvement. Advanced imaging studies are then obtained showing multiple lytic areas and pathologic fractures. He is subsequently diagnosed with multiple myeloma but cannot participate in treatment because of severe pain. He undergoes multilevel vertebral augmentation in several staged procedures. His back pain remits and he is able to undergo chemotherapy treatments and stem cell transplantation (**Figs. 13–15**).

A 26-year-old man presents to the emergency department with intractable back pain. He is hospitalized for pain control but narcotic medication is unable to control

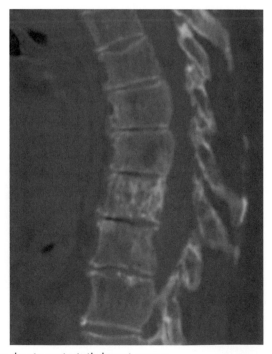

**Fig. 18.** Lytic lesion due to metastatic breast cancer.

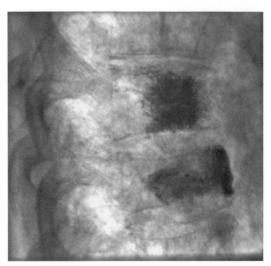

**Fig. 19.** Postvertebral augmentation.

his pain. Advanced imaging shows a midthoracic lytic lesion (**Fig. 16**). On further workup he is found to have metastatic lung cancer. He undergoes a single-level kyphoplasty with complete resolution of his pain (**Fig. 17**). He was discharged from the hospital and able to seek cancer care on an outpatient basis.

An 80-year-old woman with widely metastatic breast cancer presents to clinic with back pain (**Fig. 18**). She has strong beliefs in alternative and holistic methods of care.

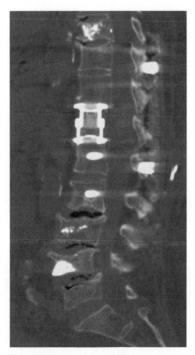

**Fig. 20.** L5 fracture in complex postoperative spine.

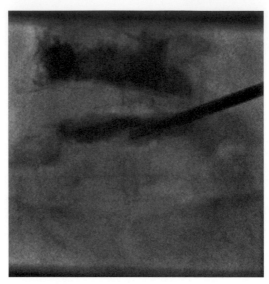

**Fig. 21.** L5 vertebroplasty.

She has declined chemotherapy and radiation treatments. She declines all narcotic pain medications. A fiercely independent woman, she only consents to the consult because the pain is limiting her ability to care for herself at home. After much discussion, she opts to undergo vertebral augmentation (**Fig. 19**). She has near-complete resolution of her pain and maintains her independence.

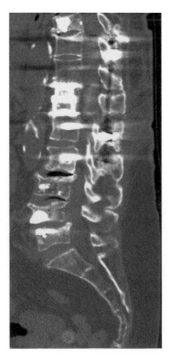

**Fig. 22.** After augmentation.

A 67-year-old woman presents to clinic with intractable back pain. Her past medical history is significant for extensive back surgery with instrumentation. Her lumbar fusion has been successful for many years. She reports a sudden increase of low-back pain without a related trauma or sentinel event. After several weeks of conservative management she undergoes advanced imaging (**Fig. 20**). An acute vertebral body compression fracture is found at L5. She undergoes successful L5 vertebral augmentation with excellent resolution of her fracture-related pain (**Figs. 21** and **22**).

## SUMMARY

Compression fractures are a common cause of pain and loss of independence. Painful vertebral body compression fractures lead to significant morbidity and mortality in the elderly and oncology patient populations. This condition relates to pulmonary dysfunction, eating disorders (nutritional deficits), pain, loss of independence, and changes in mental status related to pain and medications. Medical management has advanced in slowing the progress of osteoporosis; however, vertebral body compression fractures remain a frequent occurrence and their treatment is difficult. Vertebroplasty and kyphoplasty are percutaneous procedures and offer an attractive alternative for the treatment of compression fractures and spine metastases. They provide stabilization, pain relief, and improved physical function beyond that afforded by conservative management.

## REFERENCES

1. Miller J. Augmentation therapy for vertebral compression fractures. Radiology Rounds 2009;7:1–4.
2. National Osteoporosis Foundation. Available at: http://www.nof.org.
3. Diamond TH, Champion B, Clark WA. Management of acute osteoporotic vertebral fractures: a nonrandomized trial comparing percutaneous vertebroplasty with conservative therapy. Am J Med 2003,114:257–65.
4. Gailbert P, Deramond H, Rosat P, et al. Preliminary note on the treatment of vertebral angioma by percutaneous acrylic vertebroplasty. Neurochirurgie 1987;33: 166–8.
5. Weill A, Chiras J, Simon JM, et al. Spinal metastases: indications for and results of percutaneous injection of acrylic surgical cement. Radiology 1996;199:241–7.
6. Cotton A, Dewartre F, Cortet B, et al. Percutaneous vertebroplasty for osetolytic metastases and myeloma: effects of the percentage of lesion filling and the leakage of methyl methacrylate at clinical follow-up. Radiology 1996;200:525–30.
7. Jensen ME, Evans AJ, Mathis JM, et al. Percutaneous polymethylmethacrylate vertebroplasty in the treatment of osteoporotic vertebral body compression fractures: technical aspects. AJNR Am J Neuroradiol 1997;18:1897–904.
8. Garfin 3R, Yuan HA, Reiley MA. New technologies in spine: kyphoplasty and vertebroplasty for the treatment of painful osteoporotic compression fractures. Spine (Phila Pa 1976) 2001;26:1511–5.
9. Wardlaw D, Cummings SR, Van Meirhaeghe J, et al. Efficacy and safety of balloon kyphoplasty compared with non-surgical care for vertebral compression fracture (FREE): a randomised controlled trial. Lancet 2009;373:1016–23.
10. Anselmetti GC, Corgnier A, Debernardi F, et al. Treatment of painful compression vertebral fractures with vertebroplasty: results and complications. Radiol Med 2005;110(3):262–72.

11. Do HM, Kim BS, Marcellus ML, et al. Prospective analysis of clinical outcomes after percutaneous vertebroplasty for painful osteoporotic vertebral body fractures. AJNR Am J Neuroradiol 2005;26(7):1623–8.

12. Prather H, Van Dillen L, Metzler JP, et al. Prospective measurement of function and pain in patients with non-neoplastic compression fractures treated with vertebroplasty. J Bone Joint Surg Am 2006;88(2):334–41.

13. Singh AK, Pilgram TK, Gilula LA. Osteoporotic compression fractures: outcomes after single- versus multiple-level percutaneous vertebroplasty. Radiology 2006; 238(1):211–20.

14. Coumans JV, Reinhardt MK, Lieberman IH. Kyphoplasty for vertebral compression fractures: 1-year clinical outcomes from a prospective study. J Neurosurg 2003;99(1 Suppl):44–50.

15. Evans AJ, Jensen ME, Kip KE, et al. Vertebral compression fractures: pain reduction and improvement in functional mobility after percutaneous polymethylmethacrylate vertebroplasty retrospective report of 245 cases. Radiology 2003;226(2): 366–72.

16. Hodler J, Peck D, Gilula LA. Midterm outcome after vertebroplasty: predictive value of technical and patient-related factors. Radiology 2003;227(3):662–8.

17. Ledlie JT, Renfro M. Balloon kyphoplasty: one-year outcomes in vertebral body height restoration, chronic pain, and activity levels. J Neurosurg 2003;98:36–42.

18. Hirsch AE, Medich DC, Rosenstein BS, et al. Radioisotopes and vertebral augmentation: dosimetric analysis of a novel approach for the treatment of malignant compression fractures. Radiother Oncol 2008;87:119–26.

19. Jha RM, Yoo AJ, Hirsch AE, et al. Predictors of successful palliation of compression fractures with vertebral augmentation: single-center experience of 525 cases. J Vasc Interv Radiol 2009;20:760–8.

20. Jensen ME, McGraw JK, Cardella JF, et al. Position statement on percutaneous vertebral augmentation: a consensus statement developed by the American Society of Interventional and Therapeutic Neuroradiology, Society of Interventional Radiology, American Association of Neurological Surgeons/Congress of Neurological Surgeons, and American Society of Spine Radiology. J Vasc Interv Radiol 2007;18:325–30.

# Index

*Note:* Page numbers of article titles are in **boldface** type.

### A

### B

# Moving?

## Make sure your subscription moves with you!

To notify us of your new address, find your **Clinics Account Number** (located on your mailing label above your name), and contact customer service at:

**Email: journalscustomerservice-usa@elsevier.com**

**800-654-2452** (subscribers in the U.S. & Canada)
**314-447-8871** (subscribers outside of the U.S. & Canada)

**Fax number: 314-447-8029**

**Elsevier Health Sciences Division
Subscription Customer Service
3251 Riverport Lane
Maryland Heights, MO 63043**

*To ensure uninterrupted delivery of your subscription, please notify us at least 4 weeks in advance of move.

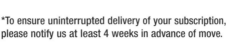